Renascent
Crystal Light Balancing
&
Chromotherapy Workbook
(Color / Colour Healing)

CRYSTAL THERAPY, CIRCULAR POLARISED LIGHT, SPIRITUAL REALMS, EMOTIONS & COLOR HEALING

By

Lesley Mitchell

Kinesiologist & Instructor, Metaphysician, Educational Kinesiology Consultant, Beauty Therapist, Gemmologist, Landscape Designer, Reiki Master, Crystal Therapist, Gem Essence Instructor & practitioner, Feng Shui Practitioner, International Lecturer & Author.

&

Denise Keele-bedford

Kinesiology Consultant & Artist,
Independent Curator, Tasun Creative Art Patron

First Published in Australia in1994
Redesigned and Reprinted in 2016 by
Renascent (Victoria, Australia)
www.renascentcollege.com

Introduction

There are many modalities of natural and alternative healing abounding these days. Some treat the physical body, others the etheric, the emotions, the mind and some the spiritual levels. Without doubt, the best form of therapy would be able to bring about healing in not one or two of these areas, but in all simultaneously.

Color healing is not only a physical force, yet also a spiritual force which embodies and includes the mind, emotions, thoughts, attitudes and all of the subtle bodies (the Etheric, Astral, Individuality/I Am). And so it forms a healing link between the physical body and the soul or the spiritual bodies.

Many orthodox forms of treatment also employ color healing (although generally in far harsher methods, such as ultra violet radiation therapy) and thus it is a possible way to build the bridge between orthodox and alternative healing and both forms of therapy.

Some patients who are more sensitive to subtle energies and will be able to feel and experience the energy flow becoming more vitalised and energy blocks actually moving and dissipating throughout their body. Others may not consciously feel nor be aware of any changes, yet the balancing will take place regardless of whether the patient can feel it or not. Gradually as the energy flow is improved throughout all of the bodies, the patient will become more aware of changes in his/her thoughts, emotions and reasoning faculties. As the negative states of thinking are cast aside the body has no choice but to allow the illnesses the body has created through these states of mind, to also be cast aside and become replaced with vitality, clarity and good health.

The three main modalities of healing are embraced in this treatment. The first being crystals, which have the abilities to cleanse and boost our entire energy field. Then through meridians and Acupressure points energy flow is improved and blockages are released and finally, color which is such an important aspect in all of our lives, there is simply no getting away from it.
When these three are harnessed together and brought into our lives they bring joy, vitality and renewed zest for life, and when it is needed - healing. Aware or unaware, visible or invisible, color and energy affect us powerfully, for in these aspects we have the true essence of our very being.

Welcome to the healing of Chromotherapy
(Color Healing)

Many years ago, I was a practicing natural therapist, specialising in Kinesiology. On average I would spend 1-1.5 hours per client to achieve the healing energies I required in my clinic. One weekend we went to a new age healing type exhibition and on one stall I was intrigued by a color puncture torch I saw. I had a look at the torch, and felt it was an interesting modality of healing, however, I felt it overwhelmingly expensive for most practitioners. It was imported from Europe and had a price tag of around AUD$1300 (in 1989 - add this up at an inflationary rate of approximately 100% or doubling every 15 years).

I wondered if it was possible to achieve a similar healing tool without the exorbitant price tag. We searched high and low for people manufacturing these or similar products any where we could, yet we turned up nothing. After 2 years of searching, we wondered if it was possible to get them manufactured ourselves. The torches themselves were no problems and it was possible to have the acrylic tips moulded, the crystals we were able to purchase from collectors. (There is a section further on as to the importance of natural crystals as opposed to cut ones and also the assistance of collected over mined).
However the colors presented the concerns. We discovered there was 57 different shades of red and only 2 would have a healing affect on the body. Working out how to determine the exact shades was a seemingly impossible task. However, just as we were about to give up, I spent the day in an Applied Kinesiology seminar and the instructor and I got to chatting about this and it turns out he has devoted a great part of his life to color therapy and has the exact list of shading for color healing which he was happy to share.
Armed with this knowledge we were able to take this to the color gel manufacturers and purchase the exact shades required for healing. These were then manufactured into the gels or color discs as we call them. In order to maintain color shade consistency it was vital that the globe of the torch did not emit a yellow hue which would affect the

shading, so we utilised halogen globes, which produce a much nearer to perfect white light and we find that the color it emits is very beneficial for healing.

Originally the Renascent Crystal Light Balancing Torches were packaged in a very basic form with hand cut foam rubber holders. They didn't look very pretty, but this certainly didn't detract from their healing abilities.

I started using the torch on myself and was delighted at the quality, the depth of healing and the sensations I experienced. After some time I began to use the torch in my clinic and was amazed to discover that I was able to access deeper subconscious states than ever before and a complete healing session was completed in about 15 minutes instead of the usual 1-1.5 hours.

This in itself posed another dilemma for me as my clinic was charged at a session rate rather than a time rate, I wrestled with the idea of receiving an hourly rate for 15 minutes work. This took some time for me to settle with until I finally came to the realisation that it was the healing the clients were paying for rather than the time it took to achieve it. If a full healing could be accomplished in 15 minutes, then that is the price it was worth. Eventuially I came to a happy medium and charged the usual clinic session price, spent 10-15 minutes chatting to find out more about the client at the beginning of the session and spent 20-30 minutes at the end, testing if there was additional foods, vitamins or supplements that they would benefit from. A lovely service that I had previously not had time to include.

After some time a few of my clients who were also practitioners asked if they could purchase a torch for their own clinics. We had a few more made and then went off using them. They also achieved wonderful results and in turn shared their results with their colleagues who also in turn called for a torch. Eventually we had to get them professionally made to keep up with the demand and the Renascent Crystal Light Balancing Torches are now sold in many Kinesiology college, Natural Health Supplies businesses and teaching institutes.

For me that is a wonderful way to get a health device marketed and utilised. There is no sales hype, no amazing promises of what this wonderful modality will do for you, many of which result in expensive purchases for items that just don't quite live up to their promises.

It is simply that the Renascent Crystal Light Balancing is a wonderful modality that achieves great results in healing, removing emotional blockages and uplifting the mind, body and soul.

I am delighted to share this wonderful form of healing, along with ancient teachings, personal anecdotes and gem essences, all terrific tools of transformation in this book with you.

Color Therapy & the 5 Elements

In this book we explore the Chinese theory of the five elements as we have found they are imperative to understanding and linking the colors with what is occurring in the person.

Originally there was only four elements as the Chinese placed themselves (the Earth element) in the centre with the Fire, Metal, Water and Wood as the surrounding elements. They saw the world surrounding them and felt they were in the middle of the universe rather than part of it.

Then they decided to focus their lives on the sun and the joy it brings. They felt they needed to be part of the cycle. To dynamically interact with the sun rather than being statically placed in the centre. Hence the people became part of the cycle of life and were able to experience the energies of the elements passing through them and bringing into their consciousness joy, sympathy, sadness, anxiety and anger, eventually returning to joy. Allowing for richness of experience and an interaction with the cosmos.

As the elements and their appropriate emotions flowed

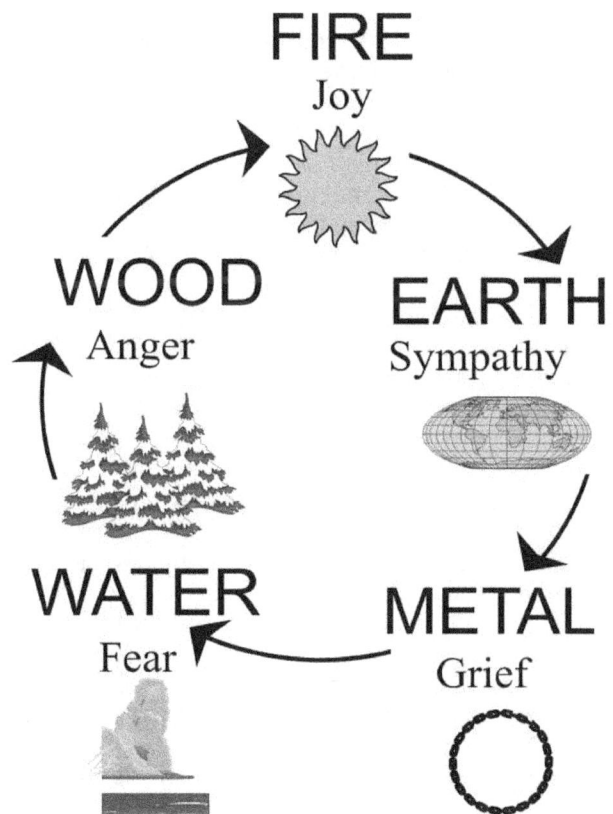

FIRE
Joy

WOOD
Anger

EARTH
Sympathy

WATER
Fear

METAL
Grief

through the consciousness of the people, this energy flow became known as Qi.
(pronounced as 'Chee') In western society it is often written as 'Chi', Qi is the traditional Chinese interpretation.

In modern society some of these emotions are perceived and yet still denied by many people. We are only now beginning to understand that in order to have a well balanced outlook that it is necessary to experience and accept all of the emotions. In denying any of these emotions the energy flow becomes blocked and we become stuck in one particular element.
Lets look at how this occurs. In the normal flow we pass quickly from one element to another, therefore none pose any problems or difficulties. However when we become stuck, for example: in the wood element, the resulting situation leads to great anger which in turn becomes a destructive force. In the same manner, we find the chronically depressed or saddened person creating an energy block preventing them from moving past the metal element. In the balancing procedure described in this book, we are able to uncover where this energy flow may have become blocked and/or stuck and thus discovered, remove the blockage and thereby produce balance once again.

Using the book without special training

This book was originally expanded from the manual for the Crystal Light Balancing Certificate Course. In order to share this exciting form of healing we have developed this book to enable you to use this modality without previous formal training and also to complement the manual given in the seminar. (Available on correspondence in 2002).

Using crystal pendulums, Renascent gem essences, colour therapy and crystal light is such a powerful form of natural healing, yet so simple, that no special skills are necessary to gain benefits from this modality. The only requirements are a willingness to learn, a commitment to practise your new skills and a desire to share your healing with others.
For those with Kinesiology skills, this may add an extra dimension or option to your balancing and we have included a section further on designed to utilise these skills.

In order to fully you to understand the importance of having an adequate energy flow and how this energy flow may become stifled, we need to also look at the information about energy flows, meridians, Acupressure points and Gem Essences. A brief understanding of the use of gem essences is given along with the healing properties of each essence. After you understand these sections you may look at the sections of colour therapy to show the characteristics of each colour and how they effect us.

The following section enables you to use your pendulum to locate and utilise the Renascent Gem Essences and your Chromotherapy torch to correct energy flow disturbances. I have included a flow chart at the back of the book to pull it all together for you.

My experience with learning any new modality (especially one of healing) is that at the beginning it all seems very confusing. There is new material, some or most of which you may never have heard of before. There are systems within systems for utilising the modality and it all seems over whelming. However, once you understand each component you practice it once or twice it all comes together easily and you wondered what it was you ever found difficult.
This is much the way it is with the Renascent Crystal Light Balancing. There is a lot of information, including Renascent Gem Essences, Chinese Philosophies, Acupressure points, Meridians, Pendulums, Kinesiology, Color Therapy and Crystals. However, if you just take your time, read through each section and you will soon see that each section makes sense and really is not that complex, then all you will have to do and make it all come together in a working order.
If this seems complex, remember you have the flow charts at the back, where you can walk through step by step in the balancing procedure. By following these charts and the appropriate reference pages in the book it will all become remarkably simple.
Many health practitioners have discovered that this procedure is vastly effective in bringing up emotional issues and healing them during the balancing, yet amazingly quick and simple once you have "got the grasp" of it.
Relax with your techniques, often when we try too hard to make something happen it becomes complex and difficult. Remember, all the techniques you will be utilising are safe, natural and in ancient times very commonplace. It is only in recent times where we have come to rely heavily on doctors to heal us and take responsibility for everything that occurs in our health state, that we have given away our personal power and forgotten the natural state of health. A state we all embraced in the past centuries.
Reclaim your personal power, delve into this fascinating form of healing and unfold the mysteries of ancient health and healing.

Formal Training

Naturally, the best form of understanding comes through sharing and experiencing hands on treatment as both a patient and a therapist. Whilst reading and practicing your knowledge through this book, will enable you to use this form of therapy, for more in depth and informative training we would recommend joining in a Renascent Crystal Light Balancing seminar. (Now available on correspondence DVD's). We also offer accredited Crystal Light Balancing Instructor Training in person once a year. Contact Renascent directly for dates. www.renascentcollege.com

In these courses we are able to share all of this basic information as well as many techniques to enable you to access a deeper level of healing. These classes incorporate muscle testing (Kinesiology) as well as utilising crystal pendulums. They are designed especially to be a fun and exciting hands on method of learning in a safe and nurturing environment. Both classes/workshops culminate in receiving a certificate of attendance, they are accredited, certified & recognised. The basic class is a pre requisite for the Renascent Gem Essence Instructor Training Seminar (qualifies the student as an accredited instructor) and is part of the Diploma of Health & Healing.

Formal Kinesiology Training

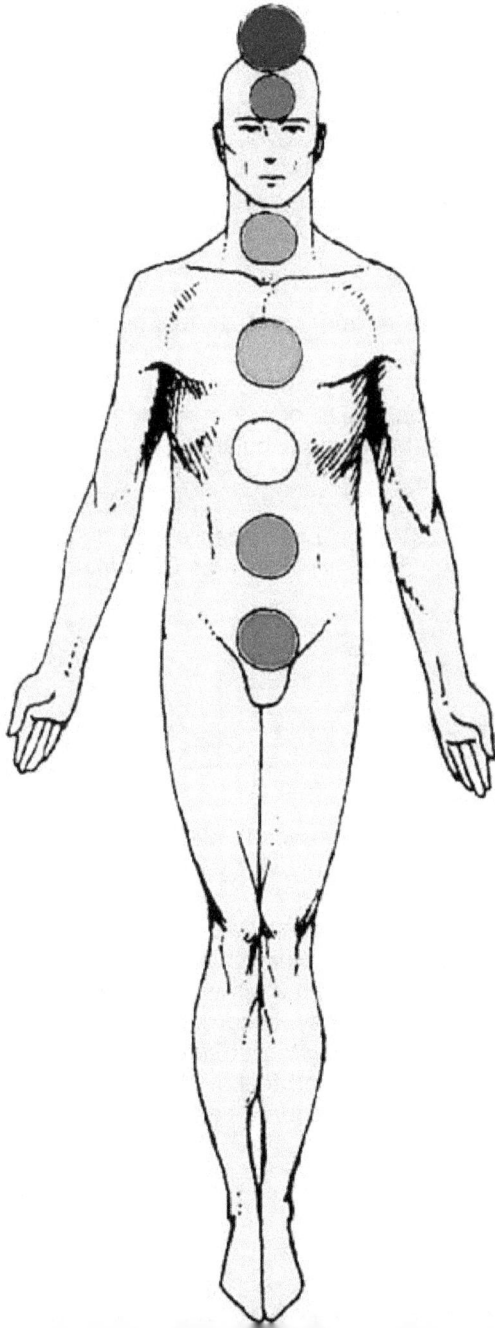

If you have qualifications and/or training in Kinesiology, you will be able to utilise this book fairly easily. Incorporating the skills you already have to locate imbalances, emotions and corrections on the body.

As we continue through the book together I will make reference to the balancing techniques utilising Pendulums (for those who desire to use them or do not have Kinesiology skills) as well as Kinesiology (for those who have these skills).

In not having Kinesiology skills it certainly does not mean that you cannot understand or utilise any of the methods or this fabulous healing. You can use pendulums and with skill they will allow you to also receive accurate results. However, if you do have these skills it will certainly add to both your Kinesiology skills as well as making this form of Renascent Crystal Light Balancing a little quicker and easier for you to use.

Meridians & Chakras

When we discuss meridians and what they are, in the beginning people may say "Well...., something to do with Chinese Medicine" or "lines on the body" or "something to do with the Yin Yang Symbol" and to a degree these are accurate. However, Meridians and Chakras are a great deal more than that and they are tangible, mapable and traceable energy divisions within the body. They are not just some vague fluffy notion. In order to understand these philosophies a little more deeply, let's discuss a little history and then some further information with illustrations.

The meridian system or Acupressure system is believed to have been developed in China. However, upon tracing this back further, the ancient Tibetans claim to have exported their art to China. Either way, it is a form of natural therapy that has been utilised for centuries. The teachings speak of a continuous flow of energy throughout the body.

In looking at Meridians we need to also look at Chakras and what they are in the body.
Chakras are basically energy centres. They are points for receiving and transmitting energy.

Most of us have seen pictures of chakras (like the one shown in the picture) which consist of dots or circle over various parts of the body and we have heard it is important to have them in balance
yet we do not really understand why or what they are. A chakra is a Sanskrit word for 'energy centre' it is a point on our body that receives and transmits energy, hence if it becomes blocked we do not receive enough energy to allow us to operate at our optimum. The resulting conditions may be general tiredness and lethargy, lack of motivation, inability to think clearly and just a general lack of 'sparkle'. The Chakra man picture shows the seven main chakras in the body and for many people this is all they are aware of. We actually have over 360 minor chakras all over the body.

These chakras are all connected by an pattern of energy lines like a grid pattern all over our body, these energy lines are called meridians and when a chakra becomes blocked, through emotional states, negative thinking, improper or impure food, water or chemical substances, there is a lack of energy throughout the entire meridian. In effect the energy is unable to get past this blockage to heal and create harmony in the rest of the body. Hence it is vitally important as you are beginning to see, that they are in fact in a healthy and balanced state.
The interesting thing about chakras is that although they do penetrate and enter the body they also exist 'outside' of the body, extending about 1 to 4 inches. The diagram here may assist to better understand this.

The entire chakra contains a number of energy 'vortices' within. These are like small funnels to carry energy in to the body and transmit used or unwanted energy back out of the body. All of the vortices in the healthy chakra rotate fairly rapidly. However through many reasons of ill health in the chakra, some of which we have previously discussed, they can become damaged. In some cases this means some or all of the vortices will slow down and may actually cease rotating in severe cases, when this occurs the entire chakra will almost close down. In other cases a single vortice may become shrivelled or withdrawn back into the chakra, or it may lose it tautness and extend out of the chakra flopping around with the rotation. Naturally we are not generally aware of this on a conscious level, yet even so the effect on our energy levels is dramatic and with the introduction of Kirlian and other such methods of observing these fields we shall surely all realise their importance. So lets look at how we go about getting the energy flowing along the meridians properly, to assist in restoring balance to all the minor chakras along that Meridian system and subsequently the entire being back into a state of good health.

Remember, the pathways this energy flows along from Chakra to Chakra are known as meridians. In this book we look at the 14 major meridians and the organs which these meridians flow energy to.

As we continue along we will learn the direction and movement of Ch'i (energy) along each of the meridians, their associated color, emotions and Renascent gem essences that assist to bring them back into a balanced state and hold the body in this state for as long as possible.

*NOTE: The twelve meridians (except Central and Governing) are bilateral (duplicated on both sides of the body) even though for clarity in drawings they are shown only once. The two remaining meridians are known as Central and Governing and run up the midline of the body.

Qi Flow ('Chi' - Chee)

The life giving energy that flows throughout the body is known as Chee (this is how it is pronounced), although it may be spelt Ch'i or Qi. This is the sustaining, healthy, energy that we all need to function, not only vitally but also in an everyday sense. As long as a person is alive there is Qi flow within the body.
Although there are many different energy pathways in the body, the Qi energy that we have been discussing, flows along the meridians. Along the meridians we also find Chakras, (as discussed), which connect the physical body, the subtle bodies and incoming energy). Most people are aware of the seven major Chakras, yet remain oblivious to the fact that we actually have over 360 different Chakras in our body. These Chakras may become blocked or imbalanced due to a number of reasons. Such examples may be stress, diet, inadequate water, structural stress - from the way we use our bodies and most often psychological stress from the way we think and feel. It is in this area that our emotions play such a large part, for often we find large energy disturbances due to energy being consumed by a negative emotion.

When these chakra points become blocked (due to whatever reason) energy is unable to flow along the meridian past this blockage. As there are numerous Chakras (energy points) along each meridian, this blockage may occur at any given point along the meridian where a chakra is located. The resulting situation is that the energy flow up to and prior to the blocked chakra flows freely, however as it is unable to get past the blockage, the remaining portion of the meridian obtains little or no energy. (In muscle testing - Kinesiology this will create an unlocking or weakened muscle)

Many people go about their day to day life completely oblivious to the fact that they may have numerous energy blockages within their body. Some of the conditions that may be created through this energy blockage are joint swelling, poor learning skills, vague pains in the body, clumsiness, impaired vision, impaired hearing and generally feeling spaced out, off centre, or tired for no reason. And so these people pay their doctor a visit and have numerous physical examinations only to find that their body is in perfect physical condition.
As their doctor is only looking for physical disturbances (of which there may not be any) the patient is declared in perfect condition. Yet still there are the vague pains and often simply a lack of motivation, vitality and no radiance.

All of these conditions may simply be caused
through lack of Qi flow in the body.

Many people have discovered that through improving their Qi flow they suddenly become more motivated, more vital, their complexion improves and they experience greater joy in their day to day life. What they have succeeded in doing is boosting the life force energy within their body and the ease with which it flows around the body.

Often people will ask whether boosting this energy can in fact cure illnesses. In order to answer this question it is necessary to look at where the illness may have originated. Those in natural healing will be well aware of the connection between imbalanced emotional states and illnesses. What has been discovered time and time again is that as we become consumed with a particular emotion we create blockages along a specific meridian which sends energy to a particular organ. The organ is then no longer receiving enough energy to enable it to function adequately. If this is only short term and through personal knowledge or assistance from a natural therapist balance is again achieved, there is no great damage. However, if this emotionally imbalanced state continues and the organ receives a lack of energy over a prolonged period of time, then there is a possibility of either illness or a disease within the organ and/or certain parts of the body. This energy concern has now become a physical problem and for most people this is the point which they would choose to seek correction.

At this point there is work that an orthodox doctor can perform (and this assistance is now imperative) The doctor may well correct the physical concern, and the concern may be permanently or temporarily healed. In so many cases, however, we find the illness or disease eventually reappears. What has occurred is that although the physical body has been treated the emotional state that ultimately leads to this condition has been ignored. The emotion (continuing to cause an energy blockage) restricts energy getting through and as the organ or physical body is still not receiving the energy necessary, over time the problem(s) recur.

A far better form of treatment would be to notice the lack of energy getting to any part of the body and work on strengthening the life force energy throughout the body before any physical damage occurs. If the lack of energy has already created an illness within the body and orthodox treatment is necessary (for the damage that has occurred) a far better cure is to utilise alternative therapy along with the orthodox treatment. As the illness/damage is corrected and healed the emotional state is also rectified and the increased flow of life force energy thus prevents future illness or disease being created, as well as ensuing good health.

In this manner you can begin to understand how this form of therapy may actually heal and assist in the prevention of illness, disease or sickness, through treating the emotional states and the energy flow. At no point are we actually working directly with an organ or an illness/disease, rather we are improving the energy flow around the body and harmonising the way the body feels about the emotional states, to enable the body to cast off the illness itself.

For surely when any part of the body becomes ill, there is a mini death occurring in some part of the person, so the only way of restoring health is by reintroducing life, life force energy to repair the damaged or injured part. This in no way can be achieved by any drug, nor poison, nor by any treatment which does not have the necessary natural elements.

Through checking the energy flow along the meridians at regular intervals or when you feel your body is not in peak condition, the blockages that you may not be aware of can be found and corrected, thereby assisting in the maintenance of a healthy well-balanced physical, emotional and spiritual body. When harmony is achieved and the physical, emotional and spiritual bodies are aligned, in accordance to Natural Law, we are able to expect a more advanced state of being and way of life.

Acupuncture Points

The minor Chakras that we have been discussing are aloso known by another term - Acupuncture Points. As you can imagine, as we are clearing the energy through the meridians we are generally clearing the minor chakras or acupuncture points along the way.

However, in some cases a specific point may have become blocked to such an extent that a general meridian clearing may not be enough to remove the imbalance. In this instance we may need to work directly with the acupuncture point that is causing the blockage or a general acupuncture point that strengthens the Qi or energy flow along the entire meridian.

Another method of allowing energy to flow through the body, as we previously mentioned is through the use of acupuncture points. These points essentially open the energy gateways to dissipate energy blockages and boost the energy flow along the meridians. Effectively clearing emotional blockages and allowing the energy to circulate and flow freely throughout the body once again.

As we continue you will learn how to correct the energy flow through the use of both the meridian itself and an associated acupuncture point for each meridian.

We will be utilising the Renascent Crystal Light Balancing torch and the appropriate color to rebalance the Qi to both the meridians and the acupuncture points. Prior to this we will be locating the emotions that have led to the imbalance being created (which will be cleared by the balancing technique). After our work has finished you may like to use the Renascent Gem Essences to strengthen your work, assist in healing the emotional blockage and laying down the foundation for solid health and harmony.

In order to understand how this occurs, let's look briefly at the use of Renascent Gem Essences.

Gem Essences

Many people have heard of and are using flower essences; the Renascent gem essences are a similar form of harnessing energies. In fact in many ways the path has been paved through using flower essences for gem essences to now be easily accepted. The difference between the flower essences and the gem essences is that flower essences work on the mental and emotional realms to create balance. Renascent gem essences work on the mental, emotional and physical realms, therefore if physical damage has taken place the best solution would be to use just gem essences or Renascent gem and flower essences (they blend perfectly together). It has also been seen with some clients that if a concern or issue has deep seated origins the gem essence seems particularly capable of delving into its roots and creating balance on a base level to dissipate the blockages creating the concern.

The essence is made to heal not an asthma or an arthritis or an ache, but to change a negative or imbalanced state of mind to a positive easy one. Banishing fear and removing anxiety, irritability and nervous tension to create self confidence, self worth, peace and strength, amongst many other qualities and therefore allowing the body to heal any illness or imbalance that may be creating disease through using a method of self healing.

The Renascent gem Essences are not a necessary aspect of this form of balancing. That is to say that without the essences a balance can still be achieved effectively. However through using the essences in combination with the balance they have the added bonus of boosting the energy through the balance and anchoring in the changes even more deeply and powerfully.

The Renascent gem Essences work to harmonise and balance the subtle bodies in a very similar way to colour therapy. Hence they are perfect companions in natural healing. In this healing procedure the Renascent gem Essences, which are listed at the bottom of each organ page, thus become optional rather than necessary. Remember though, in using the Renascent gem Essences WITH the Renascent Crystal Light Balancing they will enhance the treatment, boosting the energy and anchoring the transformation.

The essences work on an inner cellular level and vibrational structure of the body and its organs and work their way out to the outer vibrational frequency. They also work with the Pineal and Pituitary glands to refresh and revitalise the soul. This allows the essences to be more effective than physical gems and crystals, which work on the outer vibrational level coming inwards.

There are many reasons why essences assist the balance, the most easily understood is that they assist the body (on an energy level) to have a boost of healing energy when it is most needed (at the out set of the healing) and then continue to provide a strength of healing whilst the body gets used to the new state of being. In utilising the essences in this manner, the body is less likely to revert to the old (imbalanced) state which it was used to and progress (with the essence assistance) into the new revitalised healthier state of being.

Renascent Gem Essence Manufacture

For detailed information on how the Renascent Gem Essences are prepared and how to use them, read the 'Gem Essence Workbook' by Lesley Mitchell, available from Renascent and most 'New Age' stores. Some information can be found on www.renascentcollege.com under "topics". Also on www.RenascentBathBody.com.au

Further Gem Essence Information

For more information, including other varieties of essences, products and the difference between professionally manufactured gem essences and the home made variety. I have included a section at the rear of this book entitles "previously discussed topics". This should provide you with deeper awareness and insights if desired.

The following extract is reprinted with permission from Awaken Your Energies (Book)

Collected Versus Mined Crystals

Many crystals today are being mined and a huge amount of earth is being damaged and destroyed in the process in very unenvironmentally friendly ways. In Aboriginal culture the earth is viewed as the mother and to dig into her and leave her ripped apart and damaged is called 'raping of mother earth'. Although I do sometimes use mined crystals, I also prefer to have a range of collected crystals. I used to call these 'organic' crystals, although in a gemmological sense organic crystals are those which have originally come from an organic source such as Amber and Fossils. We used this term loosely as a nickname for the description of how these gems have been collected, although I now more accurately prefer to simply call them collected crystals. This means crystals which are simply picked up from the surface without large expanses of digging or heavy machinery. Thus there is no damage to mother earth, if digging does occur then it is carefully replaced and left the way it was before. I often collect my own crystals and this can be great fun. If you would like to know where you can go to collect your gems I suggest you join a gem club in your area, these are listed under Lapidary Clubs in the phone book and they often organise field trips to collection grounds as well as lots of fun get togethers with other collectors. If you simply desire to purchase the Collected crystals, Renascent has a full range of crystals and gems for wholesale and retail sales.

As you may imagine these crystals and gems are not always as spectacular as the mined variety. It is a little like comparing organic fruit to supermarket fruit. The supermarket fruit has a beautiful coating of wax, making the fruit lovely and shiny, it has also been sprayed with pesticides so it is unlikely the fruit will have blemishes from insects and often the food is color enhanced or artificially ripened. This all adds up to a lovely looking piece of fruit.

However, are you sure this is what you wish to eat and put into your body or would you prefer the unshiny, natural fruit, with no pesticides and greater life force energy that may have a couple of marks and spots as it is not treated in any way? The choice is always yours.

This is not to say that mined crystals are harmful to your health in any way - they aren't, yet they are dug up out of huge mines which in many countries decimate the earth they are on. The best way to decide what you like is to get one of each type and see which one feels right to you. I find when working with these gems and crystals it feels much more in integrity and a much more serene experience when using such crystals and gems for healing.

I often notice that when working with the energies of collected gems I feel much more grounded, environmentally aware and connected with the earth as well as with the heavens and in a meditative state I find my higher self or spirit guides communicate with me more freely and easily.

Cut or Natural Crystals

In order to perform a Renascent Crystal Light Balancing you will need a Renascent Crystal Light Balancing Torch. We will discuss these in more detail a little further on, however, the tip of the torch is a natural uncut crystal. We get some strange requests from people when ordering their torches. Some people will only want a torch where the crystal is very large, others like small crystals, some like to have fractures within them so the colors are dispersed, others like them as clean as possible so the colors are not dispersed. Generally we do our best with their requests, although the bottom line is, none of them really work any more or less effectively than the other. All will produce a wonderful Chromotherapy healing. The only thing we cannot provide is identical perfection in the crystals. As they are not man made, everything in nature is slightly different. Everything has its own slightly different appearance and characteristics that make it what it is.

People have asked "why don't you use man made cut and polished quartz and then they would all look the same ?". True, they would, however the healing properties would be vastly diminished by this choice.

Let's look at this a little more closely.

If you are getting a crystal purely for sake of holding or placing on the body, I have found that whether it is cut or polished may not make any difference at all. Ideally your gem or crystal should not be cut, creating artificial surfaces. Yet as mentioned I have found that in some cases this makes absolutely no difference. The surfaces may also be polished, enabling the user to see deep into the crystal. If you are wearing or holding your crystal then the point of it is of little importance as you will be utilising an overall general healing.

H
owever, if you are wanting to use your crystal for specific energy work, such as in the case of Renascent Crystal Light Balancing then you need to know exactly where the energy is being focused. For there is a natural energy flow that runs up the inside of your crystal (along an axis) and out through the tip. If the point has been cut, this naturally puts the tip out of alignment to the axis, thus interrupting natural energy flow. Therefore it is important to choose a natural uncut crystal when attempting an auric alignment. If your crystal has been polished, it is important that the natural shape of the crystals point be kept.

* The above extract is reprinted with permission from Awaken Your Energies (Book)

I feel very strongly that for maximum healing benefit with the Renascent Crystal Light Balancing torch that 2 aspects are necessary. The first being that the tip is a natural quartz crystal, uncut and unpolished, set in the tip of the torch in the correct direction. The second if possible, that it is better to use collected crystals for the tips of the torches, rather than the mined varieties.

The first is a preliminary prerequisite for the torches, the second, whenever we can I use collected crystals. Naturally in this case the crystals may be harder to obtain, more expensive and not as "perfect" as the mined variety. However, keep in mind it is the quality of healing the torch performs rather than how beautifully attractive the crystal tip is.

Personally, I find the collected variety far more interesting and attractive any way. Perhaps this reflects a little of my outlook on life, that I actually prefer things that are a little off beat, a bit wacky, unusual or "left of centre". I have spent much of my life trekking to out of the way countries in search of ancient ruins, silver back gorillas or untouched villages rather than on the beaches of a Club Med resort - not that that is not very pleasant also. I appreciate the subtle differences in the crystal tips, they way they all allow light and color through in slightly different ways. If you already have a torch, you may like to ponder this and have a good look at this beautiful tip, created exclusively by nature for your healing benefit.

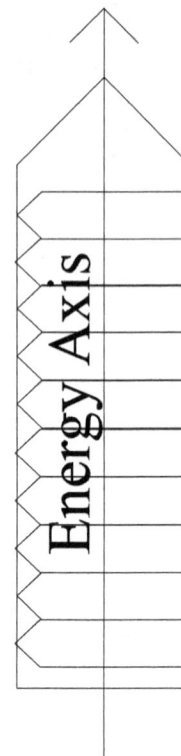

Energy Axis

Cut Crystals

Emotions

Earlier on, we briefly looked at the five elements and their emotions. You may have noticed each one had a color assigned to it. Just as each element has these colors you can see in the below drawing that each element relates to particular organs, or rather the energy flow to these organs.
Therefore the colors mentioned have the ability to balance out any imbalanced states to the appropriate organs.

For example if we discover an energy imbalance in the point that relates to Heart, we could tell that the necessary color would be red. For stomach we would use yellow. For central and governing and the metal element we simply use white light. Yet as you get to the coloring pages you will see we have chosen purple and brown to distinguish them.
These colors (purple and brown) are simply for identification purposes and white is always used for corrections. Each element also has a season and a sound it relates to which are shown on the following pages. (You will notice Central and Governing Meridians do not belong to any particular element)

The following pages show the meridians according to the color of the elements in which they reside. If you have the option of working with a partner, practice locating the meridians and running your fingers along them. For those sensitive to energy work this can produce some delightful sensations.

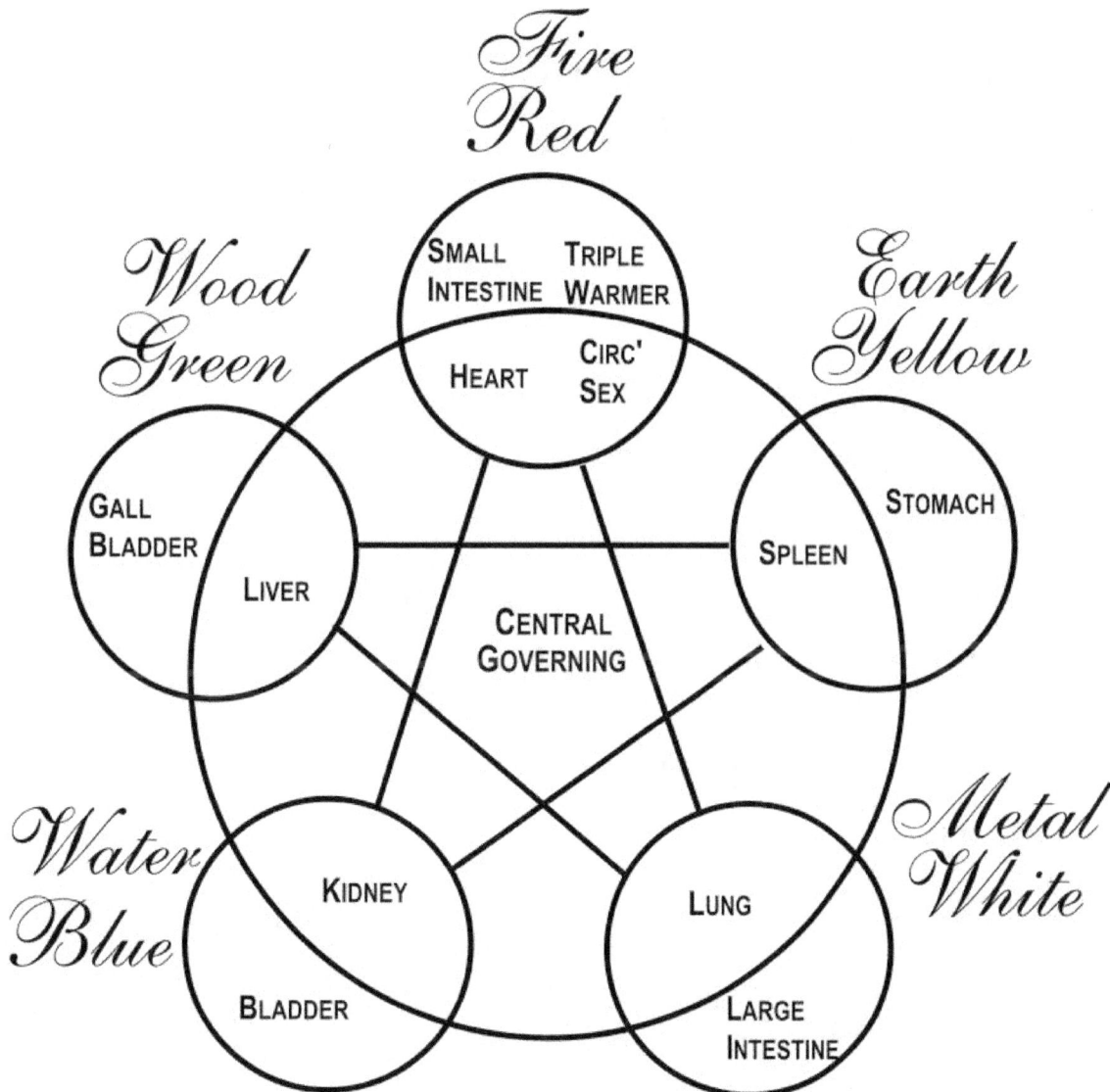

Red (Fire - Joy)

TRIPLE
WARMER

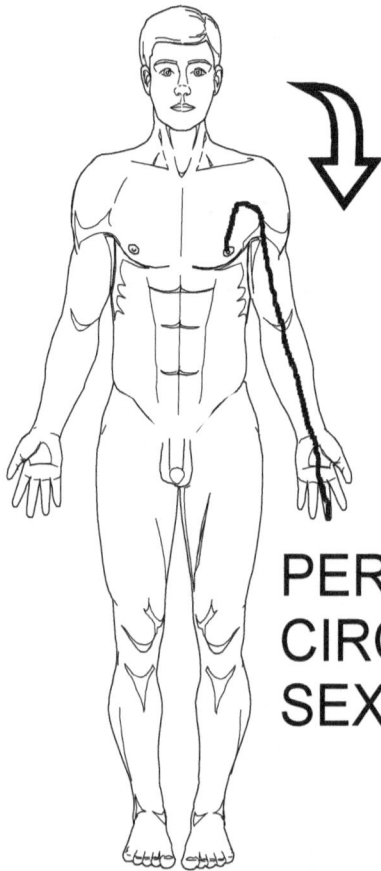

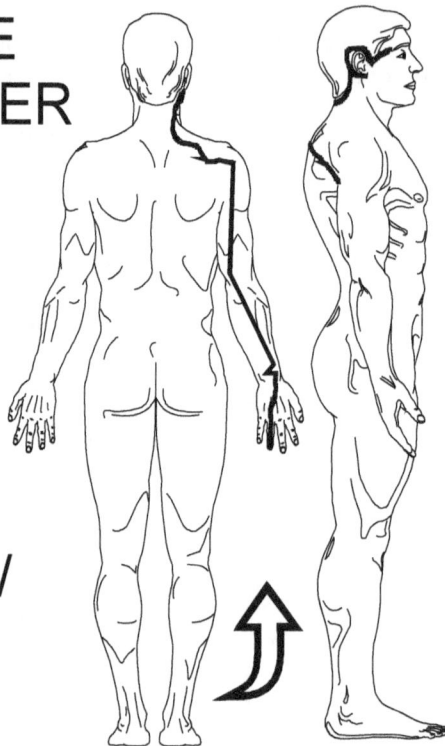

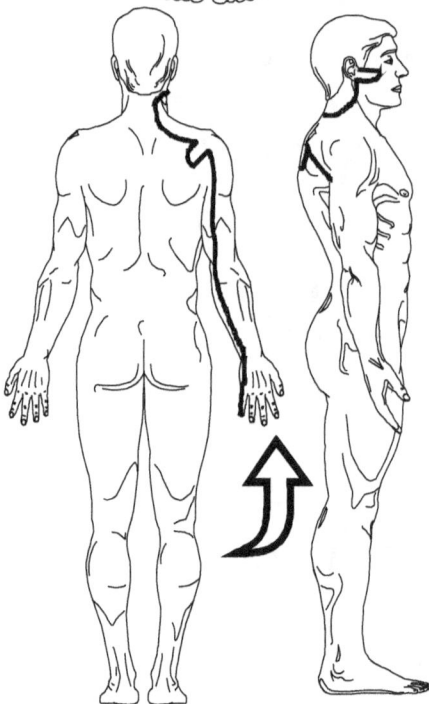

PERICARDIUM/
CIRCULATION
SEX

HEART

SMALL
INTESTINE

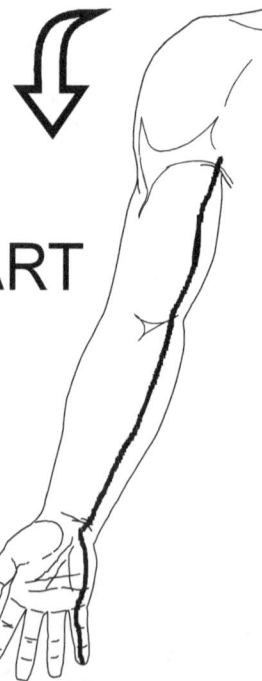

Color The Meridians Red

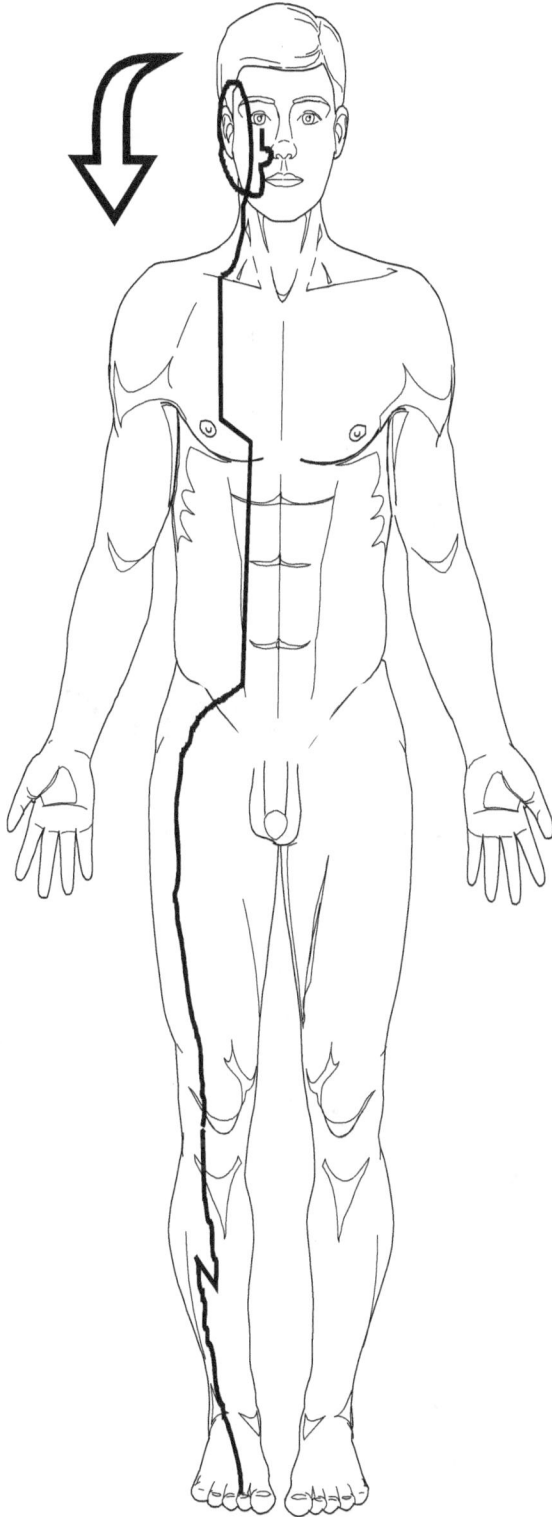

Yellow (Earth - Sympathy)

STOMACH

SPLEEN

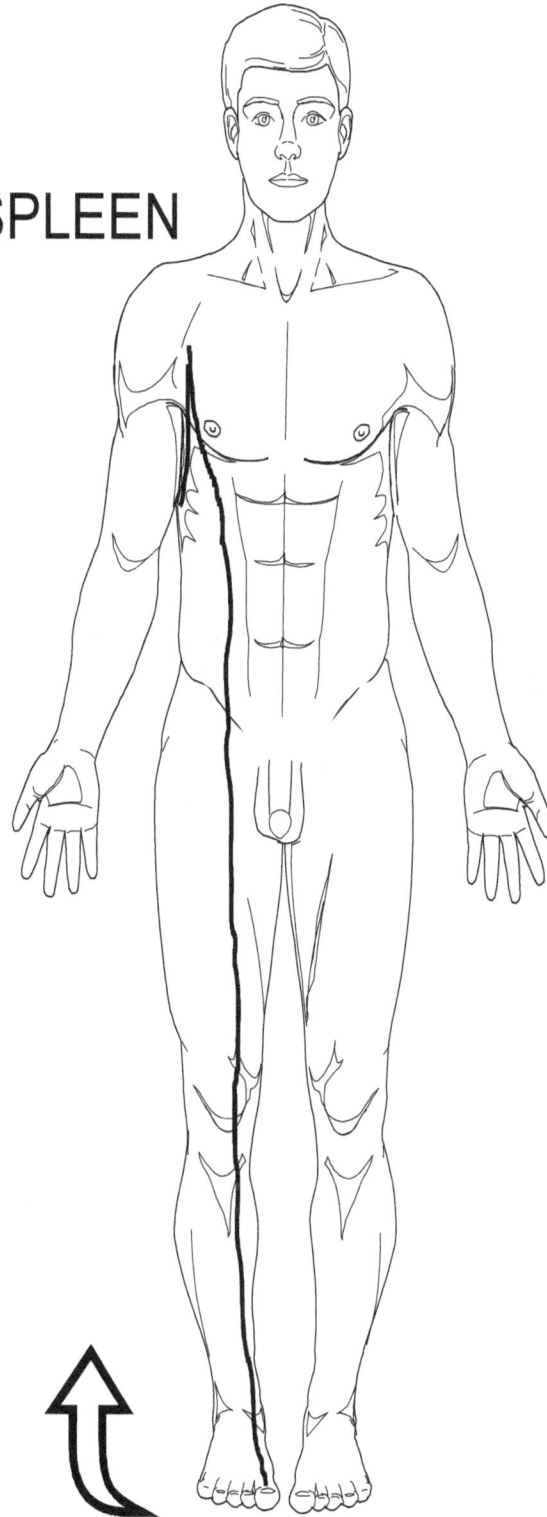

Color The Meridians Yellow

White (Metal - Grief)

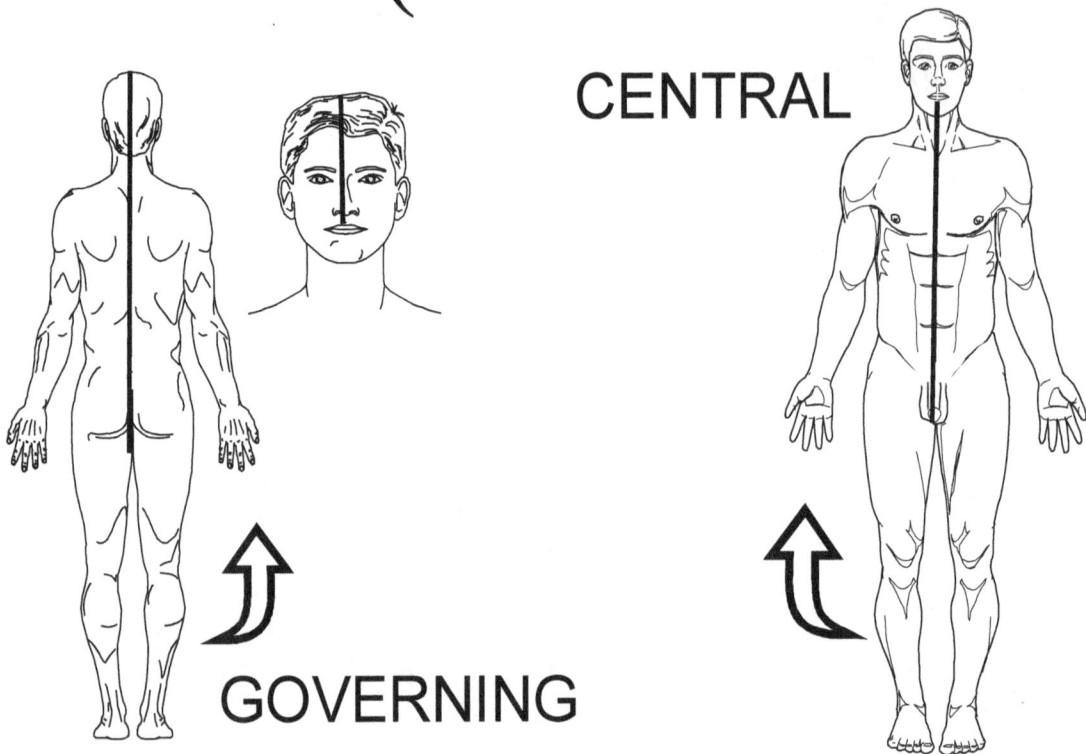

CENTRAL

GOVERNING

Color the Meridians Brown

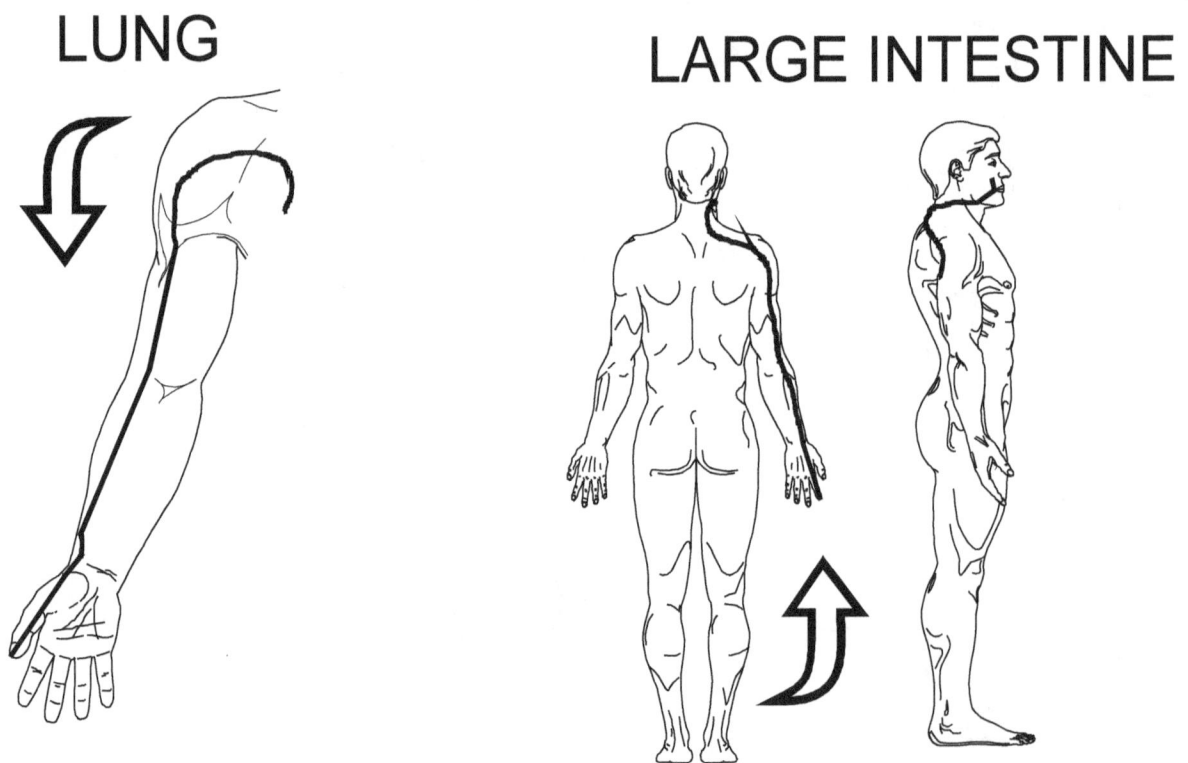

LUNG

LARGE INTESTINE

Color the Meridians Purple

14

Blue (Water - Fear)

BLADDER

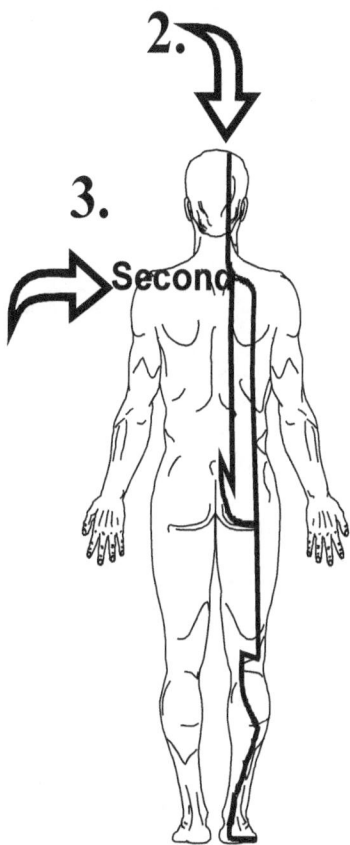

2.

3.

Second

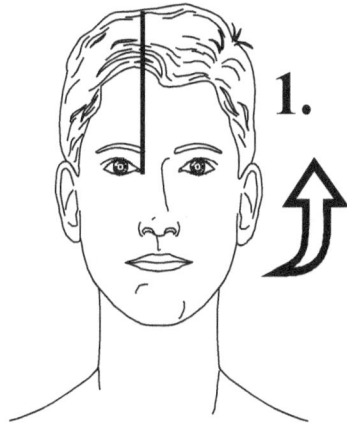

1.

KIDNEY

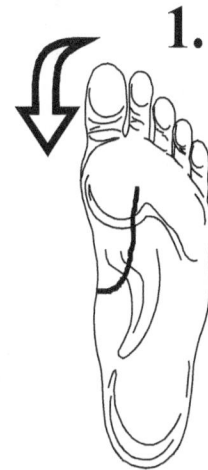

1.

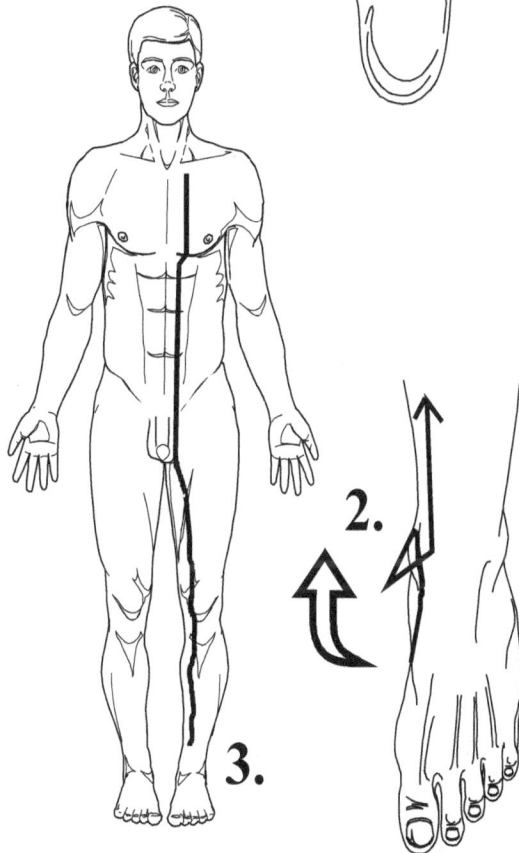

2.

3.

Color The Meridians Blue.

Green (Wood - Anger)

GALL BLADDER

LIVER

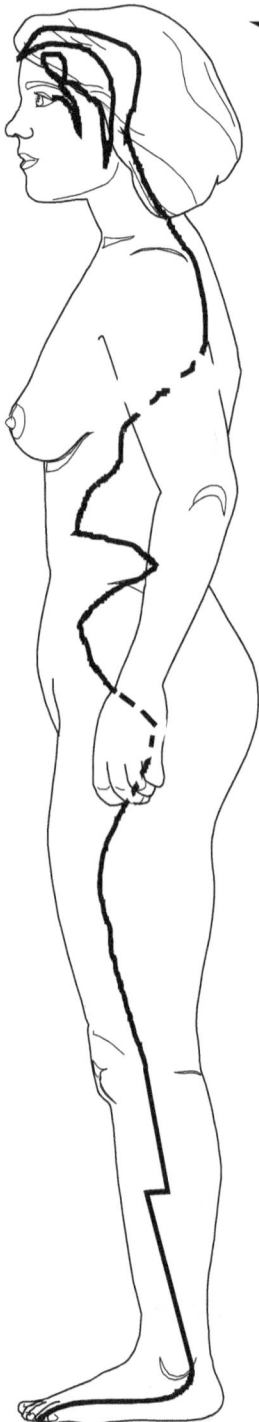

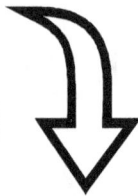

NOTE Gall Bladder meridian runs up side of body (not arm) under armpit.

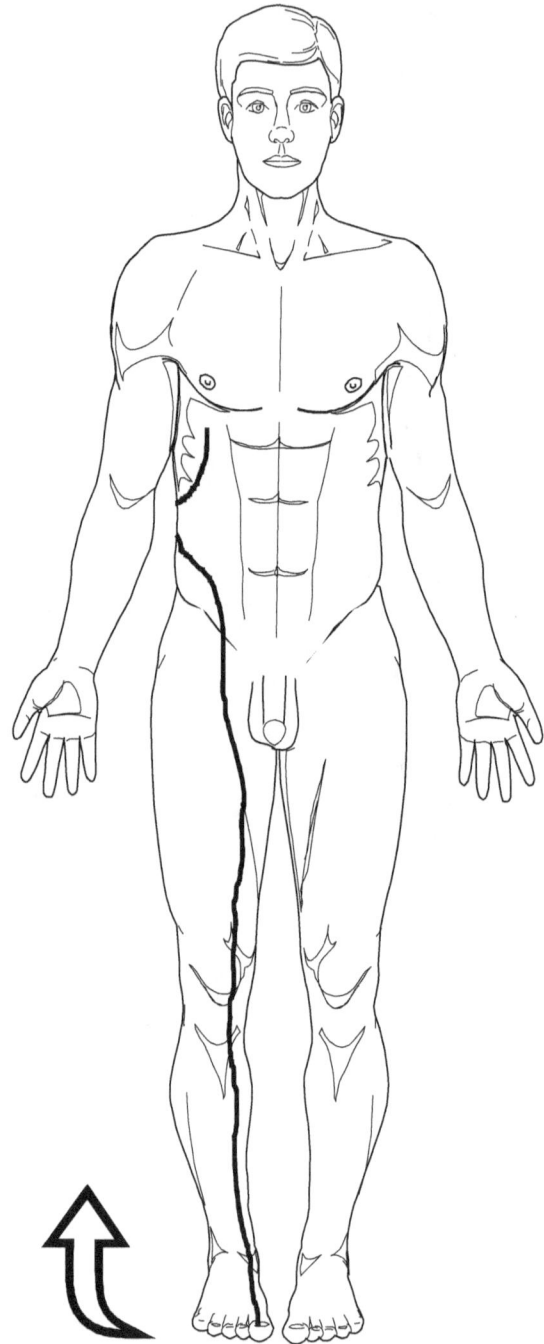

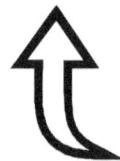

Color The Meridians Green

Chakra Balancing

Although not originally part of the Renascent Crystal Light Balancing Course, we have now included extra color discs with the torch to enable you to utilise it for rebalancing the Chakras.

Originally the torch came with 4 colors (as the tip was used with no disc for white light) to enable us to utilise the 5 element healing. However, over the years we received so many requests from people for the additional chakra colors so they could use their Renascent Crystal Light Balancing torch for Chakra balances that we eventually relented and included these extra 3 discs along with every torch set.

As you can imagine, the Chakra balance is therefore not part of the Renascent Crystal Light Balancing technique (which is entirely whole and complete as a stand alone unit). However for those who desire I will teach you here how to perform a simple Renascent Crystal Light Balancing Torch Chakra Balance.

You may like to do this AFTER your Renascent Crystal Light Balancing. If you do it beforehand you may pull meridians into balance, which if you are doing nothing else, is a good thing, however, as you will have the skills to perform a full Renascent Crystal Light Balancing, it will provide a much deeper healing modality. In performing the Renascent Crystal Light Balancing first, you will access and bring to the surface imbalanced emotions which can be worked on and healed within the session. With a Chakra balance you will be performing a healing, yet not getting down to those emotions, which, if left untreated may simply re create the concerns over time.

Once you have completed your Renascent Crystal Light Balancing, accessed and treated the emotions, utilised the Renascent Gem Essences if desired. Your healing session is now complete. Yet to make sure it is balanced on all levels, you may choose to then perform a general Chakra balance.

If this balance is not required - none of the Chakras show a unlocking response or still pendulum and you perform the balance anyway, you will be doing no harm. A Renascent Crystal Light Balancing Chakra balance will strengthen the Qi already present without creating any complications. If it is required, you will deepen the healing you have just completed, if it is not required, at the very worst you will spend a little time, giving your patient (or your self) some further time out bathed in colors.

Lets look again at the Chakra picture to ensure we know where these Chakras are located and a little bit more about them.

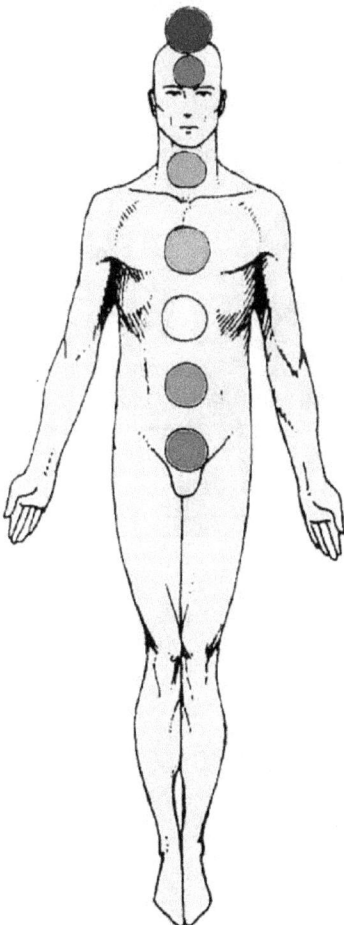

You will remember that there are 7 major chakras (as illustrated here).

Working from the bottom upwards they are as follows:

Base Chakra: Located around the groin area. ***Color***: Red.
Spleen Chakra: Located between the base Chakra and the Navel. ***Color***: Orange
Solar Plexus Chakra: Located over the Navel. ***Color***: Yellow.
Heart Chakra: Located between the nipples. ***Color***: Green.
Throat Chakra: Located at the base of the throat. ***Color***: Blue.
Third Eye Chakra: Located in the middle of the forehead. ***Color***: Violet.
Crown Chakra: Located on the top of the head. ***Color***: Indigo

I will explain a little about what may be occurring in your life and personality if each is out of balance and then show you how to correct these imbalances.

With each chakra it is important to realise that in a balanced state they each have an adequate flow of energy to them. However when one or more chakras become out of balance, the balanced energy between all chakra alters. The chakra may become weakened and leak its energy away or it may become over stimulated and draw energy away from the other chakras (major and minor) within the body and have too much energy.

As you read through the indications for each chakras imbalances it may seem as if there is a contradiction in many cases. Keep in mind that as the imbalances can be either a lack or an excess of energy, the resulting condition can be like wise affected.

As we utilise the color from the Renascent Crystal Light Balancing torch, we are bringing back a sense of harmony and balance. If the chakra contains too much energy the color ray will allow the excess to be gently dissipated. If the chakra contains too little energy the color ray will allow the energy to be drawn back in to the chakra.

In both cases restoring balance and bringing back a sense of peace, calm and equilibrium to the person being balanced.

One of the things I love about Renascent Crystal Light Balancing and the chakra balancing is that unlike many other modalities, you can easily perform a healing for yourself. You can utilise the torch over each chakra (as described a little further on) on your own without any assistance from any one else. It only takes a few minutes, it can be done every day and if it is not required will do no harm. What better way to start every day than be rebalancing the energy centres of the body. If we could all do this, surely we would have a much calmer society, with goals being accomplished easily. This would lead to a balance between work and play, greater family harmony and unity and a much more positive world.

In understanding this, whether you are a teacher, a practitioner or simply learning this modality for your own use. Take the time to show at least one other person how this balancing technique may assist them and we will have begun to heal society together. It sounds like a big ask, however, imagine if the 10 closest people to you were in a constantly balanced state. How would your relationships with them differ, what would be the out come and what if they each had their 10 closest people also ina balanced state and so on it continues. Begin today with yourself and one other person and see what happens.

Renascent Gem Essences Color Wheel

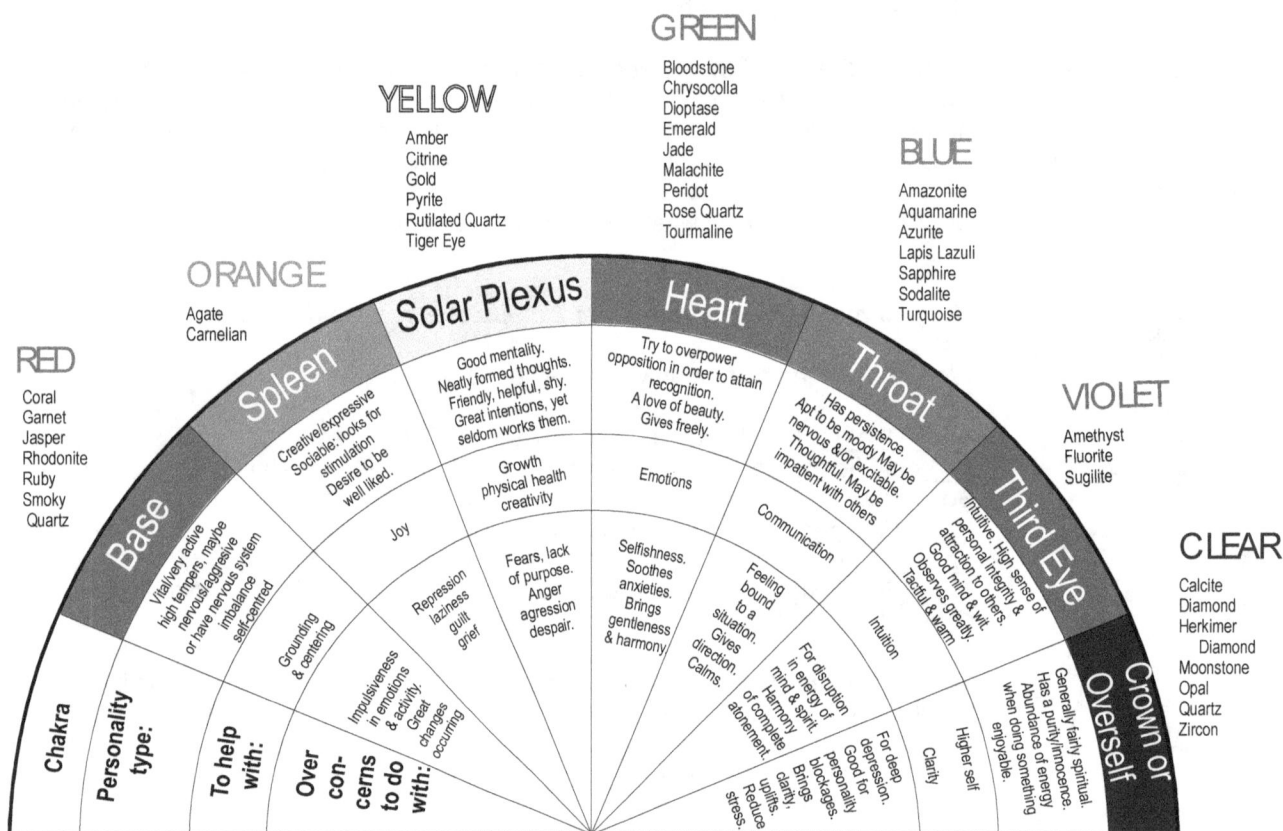

GREEN
Bloodstone
Chrysocolla
Dioptase
Emerald
Jade
Malachite
Peridot
Rose Quartz
Tourmaline

YELLOW
Amber
Citrine
Gold
Pyrite
Rutilated Quartz
Tiger Eye

BLUE
Amazonite
Aquamarine
Azurite
Lapis Lazuli
Sapphire
Sodalite
Turquoise

ORANGE
Agate
Carnelian

RED
Coral
Garnet
Jasper
Rhodonite
Ruby
Smoky
Quartz

VIOLET
Amethyst
Fluorite
Sugilite

CLEAR
Calcite
Diamond
Herkimer
Diamond
Moonstone
Opal
Quartz
Zircon

Spleen — Creative/expressive Sociable: looks for stimulation Desire to be well liked.

Solar Plexus — Good mentality. Neatly formed thoughts. Friendly, helpful, shy. Great intentions, yet seldom works them.

Heart — Try to overpower opposition in order to attain recognition. A love of beauty. Gives freely.

Throat — Has persistence. Apt to be moody May be nervous &/or excitable. Thoughtful. May be impatient with others

Third Eye — Intuitive. High sense of personal integrity & attraction to others. Good mind & wit. Observes greatly. Tactful & warm.

Base — Vitality active high tempers, maybe nervous/aggresive or have nervous system imbalance self-centred

Growth physical health creativity

Emotions

Communication

Intuition

Crown or Overself — Generally fairly spiritual. Has a purity/innocence. Abundance of energy when doing something enjoyable.

Joy

Repression laziness guilt grief

Fears, lack of purpose. Anger aggression despair.

Selfishness. Soothes anxieties. Brings gentleness & harmony

Feeling bound to a situation. Gives direction. Calms.

For disruption in energy of mind & spirit. Harmony of complete atonement.

For deep depression. Good for personality blockages. Brings clarity, uplifts. Reduce stress.

Higher self

Clarity

Chakra

Personality type:

To help with:

Over con-cerns to do with:

Grounding & centering

Impulsiveness in emotions & activity. Great changes occurring

Renascent & The International College of Intuitive Sciences - 143 Research Rd, Warrandyte, 3113 Ph: 03 9844 5888 Email: lesley@renascentcollege.com

Let us now look at the Chakras and observations of imbalances.

Red Chakra (Fiery, Grounded, Activating)

The base Chakra is imperative at the peak time of what ever we are doing, if a person is at a junction point in their life or needs to make decisions about which direction to take, this is often the chakra they are working with.

Vital and sometimes assertive - this color ray supplies our physical body with energy and vitality, the person with this energy adequately flowing will need to set goals and experience the joy of conquests. If an imbalance is present the patient may have high tempers, can be nervous or have nervous system imbalance.

Imbalance will lead the patient towards being either sluggish or over active, possibly self centered and they may have an overdose of ego at times. This person can often appear to be airy Fairy or Weak - they may not appear to be outwardly - yet underlying this there is suffering in some way which can be reflected in the nervous system.

The patient may suffer from timidness, and this color can assist to expand their mind & consciousness to other ideas & options. It is also appropriate with repression which may come about through repressing true feelings through the desire to be well liked. A lack of this energy can produce laziness, guilt & grief. Often when there are great changes occurring Eg - marriage, frequent house moving

it can lead to an imbalance in this energy, producing impulsiveness in emotions & activity.

TREATMENT: Utilising the red color rays will bring harmony and balance back to the base Chakra. This color promotes heat and an increase in the body temperatures, alleviating colds or chills, which in turn stimulates the Triple Warmer and Pericardium improving circulation within the body. It also disperses tiredness and apathy. The effect of the red ray works greatly with the nervous system to uplift, produce confidence, ambition, resourcefulness, reduce depression and stimulate activity and will power.

TO ASSIST WITH: Grounding, Centering & Joy
If You Wish to use a Renascent Gem Essence to strengthen the balance of the Base chakra: Ruby

Orange Chakra (Vital, Active, Passion)

The Spleen Chakra is found between the red and the yellow chakra. Hence it produces drive, passion and vitality, coupled with the ability to actually accomplish things and get moving. Like the Wood element, this chakra gets us going again, its energy is strongly connected with vitality and again we talk of 'getting the wind up our tail' and progressing quickly. This chakra gives us the power to get going again. An imbalance here can indicate that you are stuck in a rut when you really need to get going and move on in life. These imbalances are the standstills in life when you feel the need to create or move on, yet feel unable to do so.

This color is all about joyfulness, laughter, vitality and happiness. An imbalance here could lead to a lack of the characteristics in your life. The person with a Spleen chakra imbalance could be moody, depressed, melancholy or just generally down and lack lustre with life.

By introducing this color, the effect will be one of lifting heaviness from the soul and promoting broad spectrum energy, motivation, drive and desires. Being a blend of the red chakra, this color has the ability to inspire and stir passion within the heart and soul, yet as it also contains the refinements of the yellow chakra we find this promotes a well balanced intelligence. Hence it is unlikely these rises in passion will be that of general base desires. Rather the desires will be coupled with the knowledge of what is the best choices of action and the best method of acting on the desires. They will also be coupled with sensible thoughts. This is the best form of passion as it takes into consideration the effects of the action on everyone involved. With this chakra in balance, in an intimate relationship, there would be a meeting of the minds, hearts and souls on all level. Not merely a physical exchange.

When you are feeling lacking in motivation and drive this is the chakra to work with. It brings about the ability to become motivated again and get on with things. Sparking a creative passion to set you free again. This chakra also assists with timidness to expand the mind and the consciousness to other possibilities, ideas and options.

An imbalance shows in those who repress their real self in an attempt to have people like them. Fearing if the other people knew and really understood who they were, they would not approve. This chakra in a balanced state will assist to let go of the fear of what others think and simply be true to your own nature.

If You Wish to use a Renascent Gem Essence to strengthen the balance of the Spleen chakra: Agate

Yellow Chakra (Sunlight, Cheery)

The Solar Plexus Chakra is employed when we are in a state of thinking about life. This is a space for reflection and reconnection with the earth. An imbalance in this area can indicate that you are not using your reflective state well, often this occurs when you do not realise the need for reflection and understanding and push on in life attempting to create and build in a time that should really be best utilised for thinking.

OVER CONCERNS TO DO WITH: When the yellow ray is being utilised it produces neatly formed thoughts and good mentality. However when the Solar Plexus Chakra becomes blocked the thoughts may become rigid or tend towards lofty and unreachable dreams. The patient may appear friendly, helpful & happy, even anxious to assist the world & all people in what they (the world & its people) seem to need in their eyes. The difficulty here is that their eyes have become rigid in their outlook.
The other side of this is that this person may often have great intentions, yet seldom does anything about them. They may also experience shyness - thus they often appear to control their temper well, however they are simply more inclined to put up with people than express any great feelings about them.
The patient lacking in balance in this chakra may experience low health and appear aloof.

TREATMENT: Boosting the energy of the yellow ray can assist to promote a sense of purpose, and with adequate energy flowing the body can then regenerate cells. It can also assist to perfect emotional harmony bringing creativeness, inventiveness, constructivity, endless energy, forcefulness, powerfulness, courage, self confidence and strength of character.
This chakra cleanses the entire system, particularly the skin, where it produces a purification. This color works particularly well with any of the mental faculties and may be needed when ever the patient is devoting a great deal of energy to thinking about some or many things or situations. Treatment with this ray stimulates the logic mind and when the patient is prone to confusion through relying too greatly on the feeling level this can assist. For example, some people get so caught up in the feeling level of the plight of others that their emotions are caught up in sympathy and empathy and they are unable to do anything which may be beneficial.
For patients who feel life is rather bleak and dull, the yellow ray can produce optimism, harmony and cheerfulness.
Assists the patient with strife and self assertiveness, which is particularly important during the formative developing cycles in life.
In a physical sense this color may be necessary due to a depletion of energies that has led to nervous exhaustion, skin troubles, constipation and diabetes to produce greater energies.

TO ASSIST WITH: Growth, Physical health, Creativity   (To un-entrench)

If You Wish to use a Renascent Gem Essence to strengthen the balance of the Solar Plexus chakra I recommend: Citrine

Green Chakra (Healing, Helpful, Strong, Friendly)

The Heart Chakra gets us going again, its energy is strongly connected with the wind and we talk of 'getting the wind up our tail' and progressing quickly. This chakra gives us the power to get going again. An imbalance here can indicate that you are feeling unable to move when you really need to get going and move on in life. These imbalances are the standstills in life when you feel the need to create or move on, yet feel fearful to do so.

The Green color ray is the color of nature, balance, peace and harmony. Those with a constantly balanced heart chakra will appear strong, yet seldom dominating - these people often go into such professions as Doctors or Nurses. Generally they are helpful & trustworthy, and they may show a great love of beauty, especially song. They often have an interest in expression in beautiful ways & manners (nature, voice, song, arts)

OVER CONCERNS TO DO WITH: The heart chakra may become imbalanced through lack of love for self & others. This can create selfishness and the attitude of not wanting to do a great deal for anyone else. This imbalance is likely to be triggered through anger, rage and resentment. The patient may experience sensations of irritability and bitterness towards others. This is likely to be accompanied by a lack of contentment and they may appear constantly distressed.

TREATMENT: Utilising an adequate flow throughout the heart chakra of the green color ray provides a retreat from anxieties - it attracts & brings joyfulness, attraction, sweetness, gentleness & harmony. At the same time, the green ray acts as a peacemaker, producing soothed emotions and allows the patient to notice the   beautification of surroundings.
The introduction of this energy flow produces the experience of assisting to immunise the mental, physical & spiritual against disease.
Many people create Cancer in their body through an imbalance in the cells and on an energy level as this color produces harmony and balance it may be utilised to realign the disharmony in the malignant cells and rebalance the nervous system. (along with orthodox treatment if required)
Psychologically this color ray brings an experience of freshness, new life and brightness, as the element is Spring, it prepares the body to move into this state of new life.
Producing tranquility and self regulating emotions, this ray has an astringent sensation psychologically, cool, fresh and soothing.
When the heart chakra and the green color ray is kept active in love and faith there is an abundance of energy to the white blood cells which guard the body & keep it free from disease.

TO ASSIST WITH: Weakness & Emotions

If You Wish to use a Renascent Gem Essence to strengthen the balance of Heart chakra: Rose Quartz

Blue Chakra (Communication, will, direction, calming)

The Throat Chakra in a balanced state allows us to let go of that which we were previously preparing for. An imbalance can occur here when there is anxiety about the future and where you are headed. The Kidney energy comes into the Water element and as the Kidney holds our Qi (Life force energy) essence, when there is an imbalance in the energy getting through to the Kidney, your Chi is unable to flow easily throughout the body. This can produce an experience of 'feeling like something is dead'. Often this is a time which can indicate relationship break ups and these too may create an imbalance.
A balanced throat chakra and the blue color ray brings persistence. It produces energy to slow down and steady things. This color ray is therefore particularly good to work with the energies of infectious diseases, particularly those that have a rise in temperature. It cools and forces things to become dormant until time has passed and they can be reborn in a better state.
The person with this chakra constantly flowing harmoniously may or may not be talented, yet he/she tries. They have many heartaches and headaches, yet they will keep going in the right direction, they have a mission in life and will steadfastly go about fulfilling it. Usually spiritually minded their life is often dedicated to an unselfish cause(s).
These people express creativity, originality & individuality   (Many 'new age' people)

OVER CONCERNS TO DO WITH: When the Throat Chakra energy flow becomes blocked or imbalanced the patient can appear nervous and excitable, to the point of being impatient with others, yet may still remain thoughtful. This person will feel as though they have to meet every decision the hard way, and hence will be nervous and excitable in the process.

TREATMENT: In using the Blue ray the sensation is achieved of helping to lighten the load, and to find their way more easily. Therefore it is good for people under a lot of pressure or feeling like they are carrying a burden. This color ray may therefore assist when feeling bound to a situation, by giving direction. At the same time assisting the patient to be aware and make choices.
When this energy is flowing freely it assists with sensitivity to self & others creating a calm smoothly operating environment with no disturbing upsets. Psychologically this energy slows the mind and allows the patient to experience calmness and peace of mind, particularly when they have been through a traumatic experience and their thoughts and emotions appear to be all over the place.

TO ASSIST WITH: Communication, feeling able to cope, the ability to express yourself, freedom to flow with life.

If You Wish to use a Renascent Gem Essence to strengthen the balance of the Throat chakra: Lapis Lazuli

Violet Chakra (Connection, Peace, Balance, Insights)

The Third Eye Chakra is strongly to do with our intuition and our spiritual development. As this chakra works with intuition this is the natural way of understanding the areas involved with it. However, too often people attempt to make sense of this by rational thought. This is not possible and leads to a general build up of tension and painful pressure in the head area. This balanced chakra assists you to take a step back, look at things from a less tangible viewpoint again and relax. In this manner this chakra may assist with headaches and feelings of being overwhelmed.

This Chakra is all about spiritual connection, understanding and wisdom. An imbalance here could lead to a lack of understanding about the events that are occurring in your life. The person in need of this color ray would be experiencing a lack of connection, confusion and a bewilderment as to their purpose in life.

There may be strong feelings of depression and possibly even suicidal tendencies as there appears to be no reason for mishaps which are occurring in life or an awareness as to a higher plan. These people will have a tendency to live life the hard way and make statements like "You only live once" or "I'm here for a good time only".

There is generally a lack of consideration for others due to a feeling a lack of connection to anyone else. An imbalance can create an isolated and abrupt manner.

Hence working with this chakra will bring back a connection to divine spirit. A reason for being alive and a general consideration to all things. An understanding that we are all connected and our fellow humans and animals around us are our brothers and sisters and deserve to be treated with respect and honour.

This chakra in balance brings about broadmindedness and allows people to follow their own truth and their own path without feeling the need to convince others that their way is the right way.

This chakra is especially important to be in balance at any time you are going through a transitional time in your life, allowing you to mature gracefully, through providing a joyful and peaceful state of mind.

If You Wish to use a Renascent Gem Essence to strengthen the balance of the Third Eye chakra I recommend: Amethyst

Indigo Chakra (Creative, experience)

The Crown Chakra is employed when things are changing, in many ways this is the time when we need to let go of the old state of being and move forward into a new way. An imbalance can be created at this time due an amount of grieving as you may be experiencing a sense of loss in relinquishing an old pattern, state of being or way of life, as you move towards greater maturity.

When the Crown Chakra is in harmonious balance you will have good mental abilities with fine reasoning abilities, a well rounded personality, strength of character and good judgment. You would also have a high sense of personal integrity and attraction to others.

OVER CONCERNS TO DO WITH: When there is an imbalance in the energy to this chakra there may be an overbearing nature and tendency towards self centeredness. This can create the patient to be introspective, temperamental and generally over sensitive.

There may also be indecision, inconsistency and aloofness producing vanity and the need to revel in the admiration of others. Emotions may also become rigid.

They may experience an abundance of energy when they are doing something they enjoy, yet at others times when their task seems more of a chore they may tire extremely easily.

TREATMENT: The use of the Indigo ray brings about a strength of character that allows your patient to take on any situation they choose and cope with it extremely well, with a certain air of harmony and balance.

This color assists to bring about a joyful and peaceful kind of living that can only be understood by experiencing it. It is to do with the correlating of physical, mental and spiritual understanding. This brings about great ennobling influences, such as the ability to consider others, broad mindedness and universal consciousness that are a part of one unfoldment. In the case of deep depression, this spectrum has the ability to lift from even the seemingly most dark places and brings radiance and glow. It brings clarity in the mental, emotional and physical realms, yet it works most effectively on the spiritual.

It allows the patient to perceive things as they really are, showing up hidden reasons behind physical illnesses.

Helpful to reduce stress, this color is beneficial for inner vision and clarity and assists to shatter any blockages in the personality.

Psychologically this color clears and cleans the psychic currents of the body, if your patient has been experiencing sensations of obsession or psychosis this energy may assist.

On a physical level, when this energy is blocked the person may not be wanting to hear their conscience or the understanding that comes through enlightenment, whether this is from close associates or higher realms. This refusal to hear can often result in hearing concerns and this color ray can become a valuable tool in any ear concerns, including deafness.

TO ASSIST WITH: Intuition, connection with spirit guides, feeling empowered on your life path, finding forgiveness.

If You Wish to use a Renascent Gem Essence to strengthen the balance of the Crown chakra I recommend: Diamond

Let us now look at the colour groups in relation to imbalances in the Renascent Crystal Light Balancing system of healing utilising the healing properties of the Chinese 5 element theory:

Red

(Fiery, Grounded, Activating)

FIRE ELEMENT
The fire element is imperative at the peak time of what ever we are doing, if a person is at a junction point in their life or needs to make decisions about which direction to take, this is often the element they are working with.

SOUND: Laughter **SEASON:** Summer
ORGANS: Small Intestine, Heart, Triple Warmer & Circulation Sex (Pericardium)

Vital and sometimes assertive - this color ray supplies our physical body with energy and vitality, the person with this energy adequately flowing will need to set goals and experience the joy of conquests. If an imbalance is present the patient may have high tempers, can be nervous or have nervous system imbalance.

Imbalance will lead the patient towards being either sluggish or very active, possibly self centered and they may have an overdose of ego at times.

OVER CONCERNS TO DO WITH: Being airy Fairy or Weak - they may not appear to be outwardly - yet underlying this there is suffering in some way which can be reflected in the nervous system. The patient may suffer from timidness, and this color can assist to expand their mind & consciousness to other ideas & options. It is also appropriate with repression which may come about through repressing true feelings through the desire to be well liked. A lack of this energy can produce laziness, guilt & grief.

Often when there are great changes occurring Eg - marriage, frequent house moving it can lead to an imbalance in this energy, producing impulsiveness in emotions & activity.

TREATMENT: Utilising the red color rays will bring harmony and balance back to the energy which flows to the Small Intestine, Heart, Triple Warmer and Circulation Sex (Pericardium). This color promotes heat and an increase in the body temperatures, alleviating colds or chills, which in turn stimulates the Triple Warmer and Pericardium improving circulation within the body. It also disperses tiredness and apathy. The effect of the red ray works greatly with the nervous system to uplift, produce confidence, ambition, resourcefulness, reduce depression and stimulate activity and will power.

In a physical sense the energy of the red ray may be required in cases of anemia, poor circulation and any disorders of the blood where the vital forces have leaked out and become depleted. In the thoughts the red ray may be necessary if your patient is in state of depression, and worry.

TO ASSIST WITH: Grounding, Centering & Joy

Yellow

(Sunlight, Cheery)

EARTH ELEMENT

The Earth element is employed when we are in a state of thinking about life. This is a time for reflection and reconnection with the earth. An imbalance in this area can indicate that you are not using your reflective state well, often this occurs when you do not realise the need for reflection and understanding and push on in life attempting to create and build in this thinking time.

SOUND: Singing   **SEASON**: Indian Summer   **ORGANS**: Spleen & Stomach

OVER CONCERNS TO DO WITH: When the yellow ray is being utilised it produces neatly formed thoughts and good mentality. However when the yellow ray becomes blocked the thoughts may become rigid or tend towards lofty and unreachable dreams. The patient may appear friendly, helpful & happy, even anxious to help the world & all people in what they (the world & its people) seem to need in their eyes. The difficulty here is that their eyes have become rigid in their outlook.

The other side of this is that this person may often have great intentions, yet seldom does anything about them. They may also experience shyness - thus they often appear to control their temper well, however they are simply more inclined to put up with people than express any great feelings about them.

The patient lacking in this color may experience low health and appear aloof.

TREATMENT:

Boosting the energy of the yellow ray can assist to promote a sense of purpose, and with adequate energy flowing the body can then regenerate cells. It can also assist to perfect emotional harmony bringing creativeness, inventiveness, constructivity, endless energy, forcefulness, powerfulness, courage, self confidence and strength of character.

This ray cleanses the entire system, particularly the skin, where it produces a purification. This color works particularly well with any of the mental faculties and may be needed when ever the patient is devoting a great deal of energy to thinking about some or many things or situations. Treatment with this ray stimulates the logic mind and when the patient is prone to confusion through relying too greatly on the feeling level this can assist. For example, some people get so caught up in the feeling level of the plight of other that their emotions are caught up in sympathy and empathy and they are unable to do anything which may be beneficial.

For patients who feel life is rather bleak and dull, the yellow ray can produce optimism, harmony and cheerfulness.

Assists the patient with strife and self assertiveness, which is particularly important during the formative developing cycles in life.

In a physical sense this color may be necessary due to a depletion of energies that has led to nervous exhaustion, skin troubles, constipation and diabetes to produce greater energies.

TO ASSIST WITH: Growth, Physical health, Creativity   (To un-entrench)

White

(Creative, experience)

METAL ELEMENT

The Metal element is employed when things are changing, in many ways this is the time when we need to let go of the old state of being and move forward into a new way. An imbalance can be created at this time due an amount of grieving as you may be experiencing a sense of loss in relinquishing an old pattern, state of being or way of life, as you move towards greater maturity.

SOUND: Crying   **SEASON**: Autumn
ORGANS: Central, Governing (Not in the metal element, yet use the white ray), Large Intestine and Lung

When the Metal element is in harmonious balance you will have good mental abilities with fine reasoning abilities, a well rounded personality, strength of character and good judgment. You would also have a high sense of personal integrity and attraction to others.

OVER CONCERNS TO DO WITH: When there is an imbalance in the energy to this element there may be an overbearing nature and tendency towards self centeredness. This can create the patient to be introspective, temperamental and generally over sensitive.

There may also be indecision, inconsistency and aloofness producing vanity and the need to revel in the admiration of others. Emotions may also become rigid.

They may experience an abundance of energy when they are doing something they enjoy, yet at others times when their task seems more of a chore they may tire extremely easily.

TREATMENT: The use of the white ray brings about a strength of character that allows your patient to take on any situation they choose and cope with it extremely well, with a certain air of harmony and balance.

This color helps to bring about a joyful and peaceful kind of living that can only be understood by experiencing it. It is to do with the correlating of physical, mental and spiritual understanding. This brings about great ennobling influences, such as the ability to consider others, broad mindedness and universal consciousness that are a part of one unfoldment. In the case of deep depression, this spectrum has the ability to lift from even the seemingly most dark places and brings radiance and glow. It brings clarity in the mental, emotional and physical realms, yet it works most effectively on the spiritual.

It allows the patient to perceive things as they really are, showing up hidden reasons behind physical illnesses.

Helpful to reduce stress, this color is beneficial for inner vision and clarity and helps to shatter any blockages in the personality.

Psychologically this color clears and cleans the psychic currents of the body, if your patient has been experiencing sensations of obsession or psychosis this energy may assist.

On a physical level, when this energy is blocked the person may not be wanting to hear their conscience or the understanding that comes through enlightenment, whether this is from close associates or higher realms. This refusal to hear can often result in hearing concerns and this color ray can become a valuable tool in any ear concerns, including deafness.

TO ASSIST WITH: Intuition, control over lower, base desires, or desires of the body. Clarity with the higher self.

Blue

(Communication, will, direction, calming)

WATER ELEMENT

The Water element, coming after the Metal element allows us to let go of that which we were previously preparing for. An imbalance can occur here when there is anxiety about the future and where you are headed. The Kidney energy comes into the Water element and as the Kidney holds our Qi (Life force energy) essence, when there is an imbalance in the energy getting through to the Kidney, your Chi is unable to flow easily throughout the body. This can produce an experience of 'feeling like something is dead'. Often this is a time which can indicate relationship break ups and these too may create an imbalance.

SOUND: Groaning   **SEASON**: Winter   **ORGANS:**   Kidney, Bladder

The blue color ray brings persistence. Controlled by the Earth element the Blue or Water element produces energy to slow down and steady things. This color ray is therefore particularly good to work with the energies of infectious diseases, particularly those that have a rise in temperature. Being the Winter element, the blue energy cools and forces things to become dormant until time has passed and they can be reborn in the next element.

The person with this ray flowing harmoniously may or may not be talented, yet he/she tries. They have many heartaches and headaches, yet they will keep going in the right direction, they have a mission in life and will steadfastly go about fulfilling it. Usually spiritually minded their life is often dedicated to an unselfish cause(s).

These people express creativity, originality & individuality   (Many 'new age' people)

OVER CONCERNS TO DO WITH: When the Blue energy flow become blocked or imbalanced the patient can appear nervous and excitable, to the point of being impatient with others, yet may still remain thoughtful. This person will feel as though they have to meet every decision the hard way, and hence will be nervous and excitable in the process.

TREATMENT: In using the Blue ray the sensation is achieved of helping to lighten the load, and to find their way more easily. Therefore it is good for people under a lot of pressure or feeling like they are carrying a burden. This color ray may therefore help when feeling bound to a situation, by giving direction. At the same time assisting the patient to be aware and make choices.

When this energy is flowing freely it assists with sensitivity to themselves & others creating a calm smoothly operating environment with no disturbing upsets. Psychologically this energy slows the mind and allows the patient to experience calmness and peace of mind, particularly when they have been through a traumatic experience and their thoughts and emotions appear to be all over the place.

TO ASSIST WITH: Communication, feeling able to cope, the ability to express yourself, freedom to flow with life.

Green

(Healing, Helpful, Strong, Friendly)

WOOD ELEMENT
The Wood element gets us going again, its energy is strongly connected with the wind and we talk of 'getting the wind up our tail' and progressing quickly. This element gives us the power to get going again. An imbalance here can indicate that you are stuck in a rut when you really need to get going and move on in life. These imbalances are the standstills in life when you feel the need to create or move on, yet feel unable to do so.

SOUND: Shouting   **SEASON**: Spring   **ORGANS**: Gall Bladder, Liver

The Green color ray is the color of nature, balance, peace and harmony. Those with an adequate flow of the green color ray will appear strong, yet seldom dominating - these people often go into such professions as Doctors or Nurses. Generally they are helpful & trustworthy, and they may show a great love of beauty, especially song. They often have an interest in expression in beautiful ways & manners (nature, voice, song, arts)

OVER CONCERNS TO DO WITH: The flow of the green color ray may become imbalanced through lack of love for self & others. This can create selfishness and the attitude of not wanting to do a great deal for anyone else. This imbalance is likely to be triggered through anger, rage and resentment. The patient may experience sensations of irritability and bitterness towards others. This is likely to be accompanied by a lack of contentment and they may appear constantly distressed.

TREATMENT: Utilising an adequate flow throughout the body of the green color ray provides a retreat from anxieties - it attracts & brings joyfulness, attraction, sweetness, gentleness & harmony. At the same time, the green ray acts as a peacemaker, producing soothed emotions and allows the patient to notice the beautification of surroundings.
The introduction of this energy flow produces the experience of assisting to immunise the mental, physical & spiritual against disease.
Many people create Cancer in their body through an imbalance in the cells and on an energy level as this color produces harmony and balance it may be utilised to realign the disharmony in the malignant cells and rebalance the nervous system. (along with orthodox treatment if required)
Psychologically this color ray brings an experience of freshness, new life and brightness, as the element is Spring, it prepares the body to move into this state of new life.
Producing tranquility and self regulating emotions, this ray has an astringent sensation psychologically, cool, fresh and soothing.
When this color ray is kept active in love and faith there is an abundance of energy to the white blood cells which guard the body & keep it free from disease.

TO HELP WITH: Weakness & Emotions

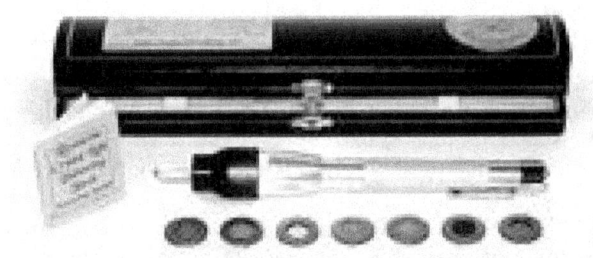

Chromotherapy (Color Healing) Torches

Now we understand the energy corrections each color ray carries, you may wonder if it is enough to simply use colored light globes or the colors in a torch. In order to understand why both the colors and the Chromotherapy torch (with the crystal Tip) are necessary, it is imperative to look at how the torches work on an energy level and the changes which take place.

When light is emitted the energy with which it moves or travels can be perceived under a device known as a polarising microscope. In a normal beam this light will appear as if flowing in a continuous stream. However when light is passed through a crystal there is a dramatic transformation of the shape in which the energy flows.
For rather than streaming out in a relatively straight line, we discover that when light hits minerals the energy flow now appears to start spinning in a kind of a beam, in a similar pattern to a tight corkscrew.
This particular process is called circular polarisation and in basic terms it means that when light is firstly passed through a crystal it is circularly polarised and begins to rotate and then spin. (See drawing)

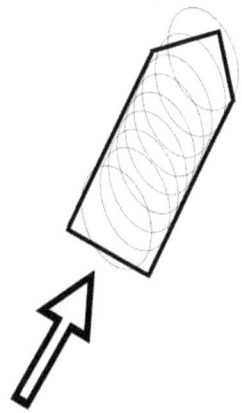

In orthodox medicine a similar procedure is utilised in laser acupuncture. The method we use, although very roughly similar in theory is a far gentler approach to this amazing form of therapy.

In working with and correcting energy flow disturbances throughout the body's meridian system and acupuncture system, we discover that sometimes it may take a great deal of time to create balance. In other cases once the balance has been achieved it may be only a matter of time before the process begins to undo itself and the negative or imbalanced state once again takes hold. There may be many reasons for this occurring, one of these may simply be that the energy was not shifted with enough strength to maintain the balanced state.
We have found when the circular polarisation of energy takes place and is then in turn passed through the meridian or the Acupressure holding point, on a energy level, it has the effect of 'sweeping up the cobwebs' and clearing out any stuck or old energy debris. Often creating balance and harmony where other methods may have failed or else taken a great length of time.

As you may now begin to see it is in this act that an extremely effective, rapid and thorough balance is able to be harnessed and utilised. Once completed it is generally only a short matter of time for the emotions to begin to shift back into a more serene and powerful nature and for the patient to begin to feel more energetic and at peace within themselves.

Utilising Your Crystal Pendulum

We are now able to understand the importance of circular polarisation and color therapy to correct imbalances. Naturally the next step is to determine how to locate these imbalances. Wishing to make this exciting form of healing available to everyone with a desire to assist themselves, we discovered a relatively simple indicator is a crystal pendulum. For those with Kinesiology skills they may choose to use muscle testing over this method, yet for those who do not yet have these skills it is necessary to understand how to use your pendulum and exactly how it works. Even for those who do work with Kinesiology, the pendulum will prove an extremely easy method in which to locate imbalances on your own body and treat yourself.

Firstly we must realise that a pendulum is simply a device used for getting information from the inner self using some type of material suspended from a chain or string. Any material with weight will do, yet the most responsive material is rock crystal.

You need to intuitively choose a crystal that seems to fit your own vibrations. The easiest way to do this is to simply choose a pendulum which you like and one which appeals to you. It may be any size, but generally smaller crystals are preferred for their ease as they swing with more freedom.

The pendulum swings through the use of the parasympathetic nervous system of the subconscious mind. These are the same muscles which direct the involuntary actions of the body, such as respiration, digestion and heartbeat.

If you wish to program your pendulum to enable you to also use it to ask questions you will need to perform the following activity. If you simply wish to use it as a balancing device as set out in this book then simply hold the chain at a comfortable height and rotate it to move in a circle, stop the swing and then hold it completely still. You have now programmed two distinct and different movement patterns into your pendulum (or rather your subconscious mind which controls the movement of the pendulum) For the procedure we are to look at, this is all that is necessary, yet as many people will desire to experiment with their pendulums we have chosen to include a section here on exactly how to program a pendulum and why it works. It is not necessary for you to perform this procedure, it is simply added as bonus information for you.

Programming Your Pendulum

You can command your crystal to move in a certain direction for you yes or no answers. Although generally people have success with the pendulum when co operation of the subconscious is requested rather than ordered. Most people will find the following procedure fairly easy and successful to follow.

Acting on the theory that most of our subconscious is a storehouse of learned memories, be they from this lifetime or otherwise. We must firstly create the experience of a moving pendulum.
Hold the chain at a comfortable height, about three - four inches from the crystal, resting the elbow on the table. Then deliberately swing the crystal in a back and forth motion. Stop it with your other hand and swing it from side to side. Again stop it and swing it in a clockwise direction. Stop it and swing in counterclockwise direction. The order here is not important, just that there are four distinct and different directions introduced for recording in the subconscious mind.

Now that your subconscious is alerted and aware of what you are talking about, you are able to question it. By asking, 'please give me a yes answer'. Wait and expect it to move in one of the four directions. When the movement has occurred you may ask each of these questions in turn:
'please give me a no answer'. 'which way will you swing for - I don't know?'', 'Which way will you swing for - I don't want to say?'. Always wait for a strong answer, then stop your crystal with a command or your hand before asking the next question. This way your subconscious has an active part in seeking out the answers you require. If you forget what a swing means simply ask again. They will always remain the same for each. Whether you ask out loud or mentally makes no difference.

As you are going within your subconscious mind, the 'I don't know' and the 'I don't want to say' can become important tools. The 'I don't know' means the answer to your question lies in another part of your mind or perhaps in the superconsciousness. In this case, ask the crystal to go to the area of your mind or even the higher consciousness where this answer may be found and bring it back to you. The 'I Don't want to say' means you have touched on a traumatic or painful memory you do not want to recall. You may be able to connect with this by asking different question relating to the original. Further difficulties may be helped by holding another crystal in the other hand. People have reported a dramatic increase in results using this method.

****

Many people use crystal pendulums to perform Chakra balances and this is another form of healing which may also interest you (for further information and directions read Improve Your Life with Crystals and Gems by Lesley Antonoff) We are using the pendulum as an indicator only to give us feedback as to what is occurring within the body. In performing a Chakra balance, the pendulum is being employed in a similar manner although in the case of the latter, once the disturbance has been indicated, the energy of the crystal pendulum is used to bring about balance. The only difference between this and the procedure we use in crystal light balancing is that we are using the pendulum as an indicator of energy imbalances only. The corrections are done through the Chromotherapy torches, utilising the spiraled energy of the light boosted by the amplified energy of the crystal and of course the appropriate color therapy.

Chakra balances have been performed for years now and it is worth understanding that there are many schools of thought over exactly what a crystal pendulum should do when a chakra balance is being performed. Some believe the pendulum will swing in a circle to indicate the chakra is out of balance and stay perfectly still when it is in balance. Others say the opposite, that it will stay still when the chakra is out of balance as this indicates the chakra is not rotating, then as it comes into balance and the chakra begins to turn and speed up again, it will take the crystal with the swing of the energy as an indication that the chakra is back in balance. This method now seems to hold more relevance for our understanding. However, it must be pointed out that the crystal is simply directing a little extra energy into the chakra to assist in improving its well being and other than that is simply an indicator to allow us to know when our task is completed.

Therefore, it is important to have a clear mental picture as to what you are wanting to occur, for your crystal will respond in which ever way you desire it to. In Kinesiology we have a saying that says 'where thought goes, energy flows' and this is important to remember here. If you ask your crystal to stay still when the chakra is in balance then that is what will occur, if you want it to swing wildly with the rotation of the chakra then that also is what will occur. Remember it is an indicator to give you answers or feedback on what is occurring within the body.

* As long as one person involved has a fair idea of what they are expecting to occur, the indicator will respond appropriately to the energy flow in the area. If the patient is not sure of what is supposed to occur, this should make little or no difference to the outcome. As long as the therapist is has a clear mental intention, the answers and responses will remain accurate.

*Remember, using a pendulum may take some practice. The more you become in tune with using this subtle energy, the quicker and more accurate your results will be.

Certain people have worked on themselves and raised their vibratory level to such an extent that they are able to physically or psychically see energy flow blockages and disturbances in the body. For these people the pendulum would become an unnecessary part of the crystal light balancing, an indicator is simply not necessary for those who can see these blockages. Yet, for the general population such subtle disturbances are relatively difficult to perceive, hence the indicator is a vital instrument.

Emotions

As previously discussed, when we deny or refuse to accept emotions we may become stuck in one element. The emotion has effectively created a blockage or a lack of energy flowing through a meridian. As in any form of maintaining balance a centre point is necessary to achieve. Imbalance occurs when we swing too far to one end of the other.

For example, complete denial of an emotion creates a situation of blocked suppression. On the other end of the scale an overindulgence in any emotion also creates as energy blockage. The person is so consumed with this emotion that their energies become so focused that they are unable to move out of the emotion. It has been discovered that each organ has a general set of emotions that relate to the organ and each other. When a person becomes stuck on one or more of these emotions the result is a blockage of the energy flow to the particular organ. This we say that the person is stuck in the element where we find that organ.

When we are able to pinpoint the exact emotions(s) causing the blockage, we are requesting the mind to focus on where the energy concern or blockage is originating. We are in effect bringing the troubled emotion from the subconscious mind into the conscious mind. Allowing the mind to focus on where we mostly need assistance and thus alleviating the troubled emotional state. By focusing consciously on the emotion, the mind is forced to lift to a higher state of consciousness. Therefore bringing the body back to the centre point of balance and allowing the flow of energy to continue. With every emotional flow disturbance there is always an emotional aspect. In focusing on the emotion you are creating a much deeper and more powerful form of healing.

*A little further on, there is a complete listing of the emotions relevant for each organ.

Corrections

We previously looked at how to program a pendulum. This pendulum is now to become our device to locate imbalances. It is important to realise that it is not a correction, simply an indicator of the energy disruptions. After locating the imbalance it is then necessary to perform the corrections using the CHROMOTHERAPY TORCH (and the essences if desired).

We have looked at where to find the meridians in the body. In the following pages you will find one page dedicated to each organ, its colour element relationship, Acupressure points and the appropriate emotions. In order to make your references easier there are 2 illustrations following these pages with all of the meridian checking points on one diagram and then all of the acupressure holding points on the second. The format is laid out in this way to enable you to go through each organ one at a time, performing corrections whenever necessary. However once you become more adept at using this method, you may choose to simply go to the diagram charts and zip through these points, referring to the individual organ pages only when a correction is necessary.

Beginning with the Central and Governing, continue on to the heart meridian (the first organ in the fire element) and then the pages follow through in order of the elements.

Central and Governing are always checked first as these are the main controllers of the body and without these in correct functioning order it is difficult to obtain reliable responses for any other organs.

For Practitioners utilising Pendulums

Hold your pendulum over the ending of the meridian for the first organ (Central). If the pendulum begins to rotate and/or move, this indicates that there is energy flowing around and through this meridian. Hence it has no energy blockages and you may continue on. However, if the pendulum remains still, this indicates that there is a lack of energy flowing through the meridian and a correction is necessary. (the end is used, rather than the beginning, as blockages could occur any where along the meridian, the beginning could well still have an abundance of energy. Yet if checked further along at the ending, there would most definitely be a lack in energy if there was any blockages or energy disturbances any where along the meridian)

In order to add power to our balance when you find an energy blockage, have your patient state each emotion while you hold the pendulum. The pendulum will either move or stay still for each emotion. The emotions causing the pendulum to remain still indicate that there is a lack of energy flow around this emotion, which therefore is contributing to the energy blockage.

Continue through all of the emotions (there may be more than one creating this concern). IT IS A GOOD IDEA TO TAKE NOTE OF THESE AS THERE MAY BE MANY.

Make sure that you allow sufficient time between each stated emotion for a response, remembering it may take a little practice to become adept with your pendulum.

Place the appropriate colour disc in your CHROMOTHERAPY TORCH, for example: if you had an indication that there was a lack of energy in the heart meridian (through your pendulum remaining still) as the heart meridian is in the fire element and the colour is red, so you would place the red disc in your torch. Slowly run this coloured light (with the tip of the crystal gently touching the body) along the length of the meridian, from the beginning point to the end. As the meridian is an energy pathway, this energy flows within one to three centimeters of the physical body. Even if your torch is above the body or slightly to one side of the meridian, as long as it is within this distance, the energy flow will still be corrected.

Once you have completed this procedure, take your CRYSTAL PENDULUM back to the beginning of the meridian, where it should now rotate, indicating an improved energy flow. If it continues to remain still repeat the colour run with the torch. Once you obtain this flow have the patient again state the emotions which had a lack of energy flow, these will all now be back in balance, indicated by a rotating pendulum.

The meridian flow has now been rebalanced, for this organ, the next step is to check the Acupressure point. Generally, when the same meridian has been balanced there will be no energy flow disturbance in the Acupressure point. Although, for deep seated concerns both may be out of balance. Generally though, you are more likely to have an energy imbalance in the Acupressure point when the meridian has shown to be in balance. This is because the body is preferring one method of treatment.

To check the Acupressure point, simply hold the pendulum over the point. Again a movement indicates a flow of energy, a stillness indicates energy lack.

When the pendulum stays still, find the appropriate emotion(s) and again using the appropriate colour disc in the torch, direct the point of the crystal on the Chromotherapy Torch into the Acupressure point for THIRTY TO SIXTY SECONDS. Using your pendulum, recheck the Acupressure point and the emotions. If this continues to show an imbalance, then the body may simply need a greater length of colour light.

* Remember that meridian and acupressure points are bilateral - that is, they occur on both sides of the body, always correct both meridians and both acupressure points when performing a correction.

You may wish to use essences after each meridian or Acupressure point correction.

Hold the appropriate bottle of essence on the cheek of the client. Whilst doing this, holding the pendulum in the opposite hand, check for responses. (the pendulum does not need to be over any specific point on the body)

A stillness again indicates a lack of energy, implying a need for the essence to be utilised or taken. This has the effect of boosting and solidifying the correction already done. In order to use the essence they may be taken in two ways.

The first method involves placing a drop of essence at the navel and then gently tapping around this twenty-five times. As the navel is the placement of the Solar Plexus Chakra (the main seat of our emotions) this technique allows us to gather the emotions together and as the umbilical cord was the source of nourishment in the womb it remains to be a source of spiritual nourishment. In this manner we are able to be nourished by these emotions and assimilate them back into a working order.

The second method consists of placing a few drops under the tongue, warming to body temperature, then swallowing. Use your pendulum over the navel and the lips to indicate where the flow of energy is most necessary. This would again be shown by a stillness in the pendulum, indicating a lack of energy flow at that point..

Using this process continue through the elements/colour groups until all meridians and Acupressure points have been checked and balanced where necessary.

For Practitioners utilising Kinesiology

Begin by getting an accurate indicator muscle to lock (Anterior Deltoid is often a good one to use) Touch the ending of the meridian for the first organ (Central) and re check. *Note - when touching any part of the body it is important to use a neutral touch i.e. the first and second fingers together to avoid any confusion in the body circuitry. If the indicator locks, this indicates that there is energy flowing around and through this meridian. Hence it has no energy blockages and you may continue on. However, if the indicator muscle unlocks, this indicates that there is a lack of energy flowing through the meridian and a correction is necessary.

In order to add power to our balance have your patient state each emotion while you recheck the indicator. The muscle will either lock or unlock for each emotion. The emotions causing the indicator to unlock indicate that there is a lack of energy flow around this emotion, which therefore is contributing to the energy blockage.

Continue through all of the emotions (there may be more than one creating this concern). IT IS A GOOD IDEA TO TAKE NOTE OF THESE AS THERE MAY BE MANY.

Place the appropriate colour disc in your CHROMOTHERAPY TORCH, for example: the heart meridian is in the fire element and the colour is red, so you would place the red disc in your torch. Slowly run this coloured light (with the tip of the crystal gently touching the body) along the length of the meridian, from the beginning point. As the meridian is an energy pathway, this energy flows within one to three centimeters of the physical body. Even if your torch is above the body or slightly to one side of the meridian, as long as it is within this distance, the energy flow will still be corrected.

Once you have completed this procedure, touch the ending of the meridian and recheck, the muscle which should now lock indicating an improved energy flow. If it continues to unlock repeat the colour run with the chromotherapy torch.

Once you obtain this flow have the patient again state the emotions which had a lack of energy flow, these will all now be back in balance, indicated by a locking muscle.

The meridian flow has now been rebalanced, the next step is to check the Acupressure point. Generally, when the same meridian has been balanced there will be no energy flow disturbance in the Acupressure point. Although, for deep seated concerns both may be out of balance. Generally though, you are more likely to have an energy imbalance in the Acupressure point when the meridian has shown to be in balance. This is because the body is preferring one method of treatment.

To check the Acupressure point, simply touch the point. Again a locking muscle indicates a flow of energy, an unlock indicates energy lack.

When the muscle unlocks, find the appropriate emotion(s) and again using the appropriate colour disc in the torch, direct the point of the crystal on the Chromotherapy Torch into the Acupressure point for THIRTY TO SIXTY SECONDS. Using a muscle test, recheck the Acupressure point and the emotions. If this continues to show an imbalance, then the body may simply need a greater length of colour light.

You may wish to use essences after each meridian or Acupressure point correction.

Hold the appropriate bottle of essence on the cheek of the client. Whilst doing this, using an accurate indicator muscle, check for responses.

An unlock, again indicates a lack of energy, implying a need for the essence to be utilised or taken. This has the effect of boosting and solidifying the correction already done.

You need to look for an unlock, rather than a locking muscle due to the fact that the body is already in a balanced state, hence you are likely to find the muscles in a locking position. Therefore in order to find out extra information, such as whether or not an essence should be taken, you will need to obtain a change in the indicator. If the muscle changes from a lock to an unlock then the body has shown a change in response to the essence implying it would be necessary. If the muscle stays locked (no change) then the body is showing that there would be no change in the state of balance through taking the essences, hence it is not necessary)

If you have received a change in the indicator muscle, in order to use the essence they may be taken in two ways.

The first method involves placing a drop of essence at the navel and then gently tapping around this twenty-five times. As the navel is the placement of the Solar Plexus Chakra (the main seat of our emotions) this technique allows us to gather the emotions together and as the umbilical cord was the source of nourishment in the womb it remains to be a source of spiritual nourishment. In this manner we are able to be nourished by these emotions and assimilate them back into a working order.

The second method consists of placing a few drops under the tongue, warming to body temperature, then swallowing. Using a neutral touch over the navel and the lips, you can then muscle test to indicate where the flow of energy is most necessary. This would again be shown by an unlock in the muscle test, indicating a lack of energy flow at that point.

Using this process continue through the elements/colour groups until all meridians and Acupressure points have been checked and balanced where necessary.

NOTE When checking for meridian and acupressure point imbalances (no matter which method you are using to locate them) you will discover that for some organs the meridian ending and the acupressure point are located in the same place. It is important to remember that the pendulum or an unlocking muscle are simply indicators and the saying of 'where thought goes, energy flows'. Be clear in your mind whether it is the meridian or the acupressure point that you are checking the response for and your answers will be equally clear.

****

The body is now in a balanced state and in time your patient is likely to feel refreshed, relaxed and renewed.

Naturally it is possible that outside influences can shorten the length of time this balance may hold for. However, the more regularly the procedure is repeated, the longer the effectiveness of the balance becomes, and the less likely other influences will affect the state of balance.

A client once explained to me how they perceived it in relation to playing a sport. They continued on to say that if you wish to excel it is simply not good enough to go to training once and then expect to never have to go again. For sports people dedicated to improving themselves they will constantly train and improve their performance, each time getting better, stronger and more advanced. And so was the similarity for this client with their crystal light balance, once is terrific, yet for those dedicated to improving and advancing themselves, the more often the have a balance the better the state in which they live and the longer the benefits are maintained in the body. For most imbalances once may be all that is necessary, however being emotional human beings, if you are to cast your mind to the emotions that constantly flood through your body you will realise there are indeed many opportunities for corrections in our day to day lives.

RECEIVE A CRYSTAL LIGHT BALANCE AS OFTEN AS POSSIBLE.

In these times of rapid change, our rates of vibrations are constantly being lifted and challenged. Many people are becoming confused and unfocused due to the swiftness of these changes. In rebalancing the energy flow throughout the body we are better prepared to keep up with these changes. In maintaining balance we are able to remain peaceful and harmonious, even in troubled times. SHARE YOUR HEALING. In working with this modality the rewards are excellent, yet in sharing your healing with unconditional love the rewards are literally out of this world.

White Central

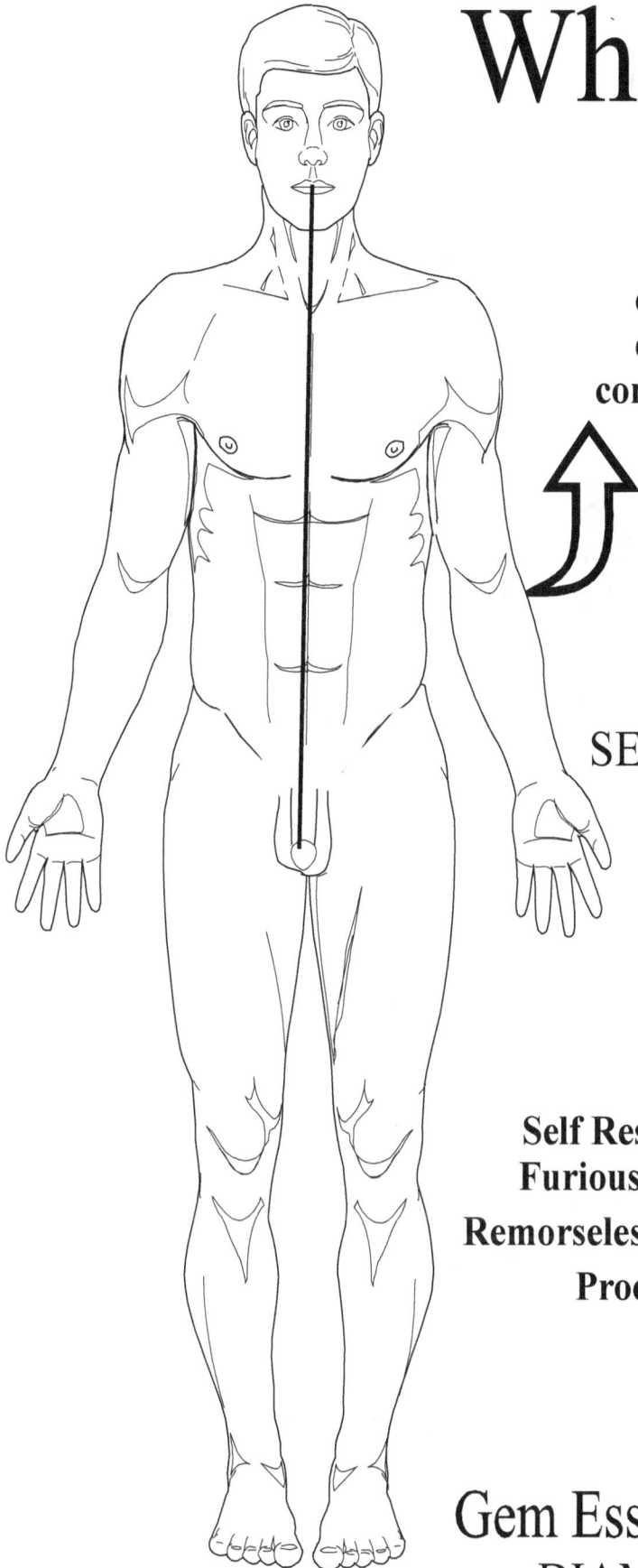

Energy imbalance may be
created through Matters of
emotion, as this is the main
controller of the bodys emotions

⇧

Spiritual Emotion:
SELF EMPOWERMENT

Emotions:
**Self Respect, Insufficient, Over whelm,
Furious, Inadequate, Success, Careless,
Remorseless, Distrustful, Boisterous, Euphoric,
Procrastinating, Cruel, Pestered.**

Gem Essences:
DIAMOND, MALACHITE

Color the Meridian Brown (White Disc)

White

Governing

Energy imbalance may be created through Physical disturbance, as this meridian controls the body and effects the body physically.

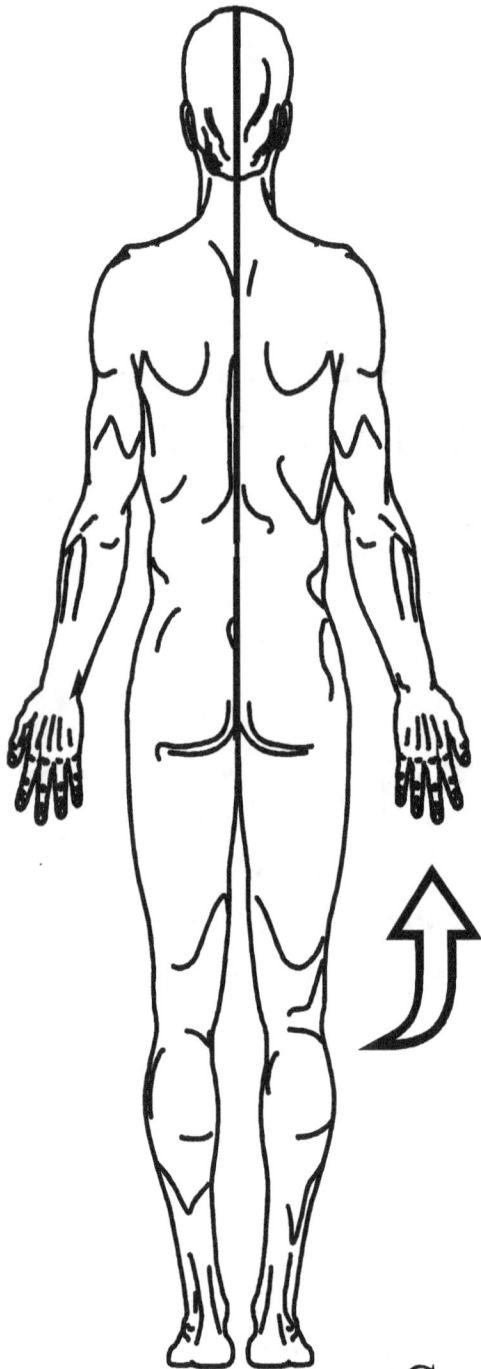

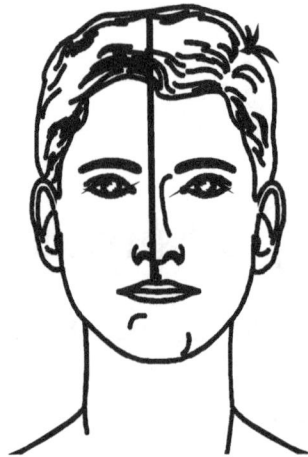

Spiritual Emotion:
INNER
CONNECTION

Emotions:

Embarrassment, Aloof, Dishonesty, Talkative, Truth, Imposed Upon, Lonely, Futile, Unloved, Haughty, Over bearing, Unneeded, Agitated.

Gem Essence: TOURMALINE

Color the Meridian Brown (White Disc)

Red

Small Intestine

Energy imbalance may be created through Past Shock.

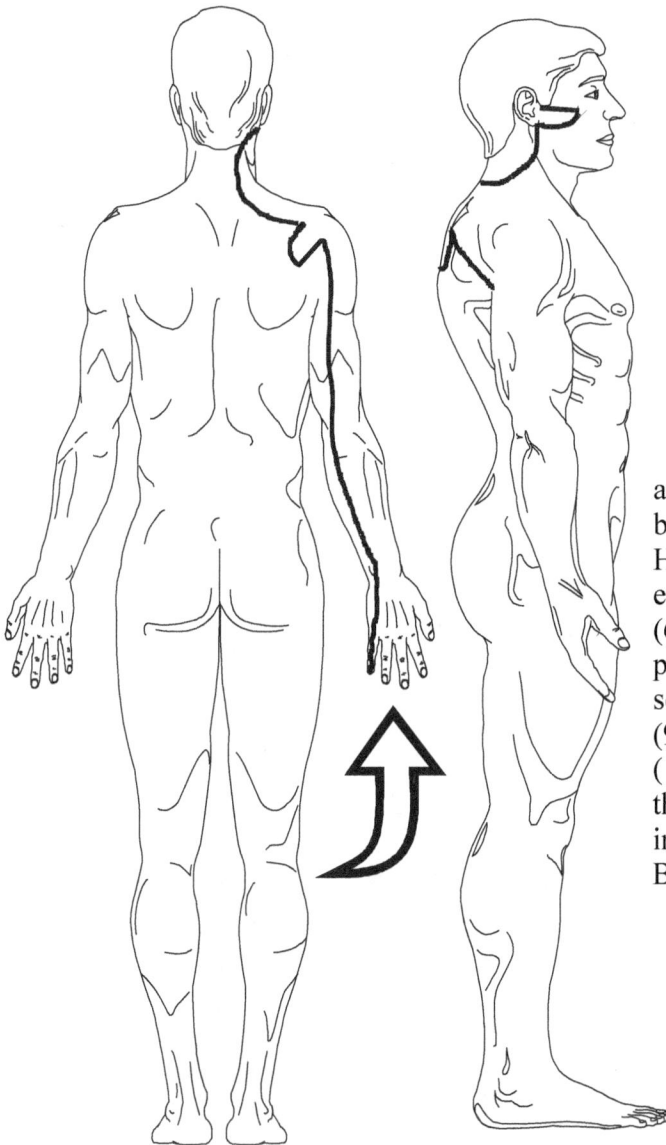

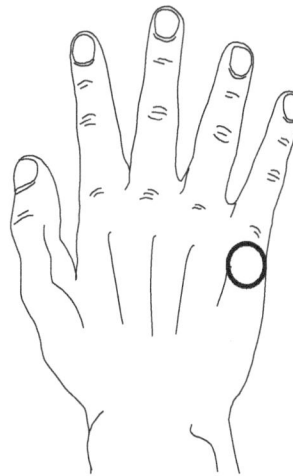

The Small Intestine Meridian begins on the outside of the tip of the little finger, crosses the palm and wrist (1), and passes upward along the posterior aspect of the forearm (2). The Meridian continues upward along the posterior border of the lateral aspect of the upper arm(3), circles behind the shoulder (4), and runs to the center of the uppermost part of the back (where it meets the Governing Meridian). Here, the Meridian divides into two branches, one entering internally (5) to connect with the Heart (6), diaphragm, and Stomach(7), before entering its pertaining Organ, the Small Intestine (8). The second branch ascends along the side of the neck (9) to the cheek (10) and outer corner of the eye (11) before entering the ear. A short branch leaves the Meridian on the cheek (12) and runs to the inner corner of the eye, where it connects with the Bladder Meridian.

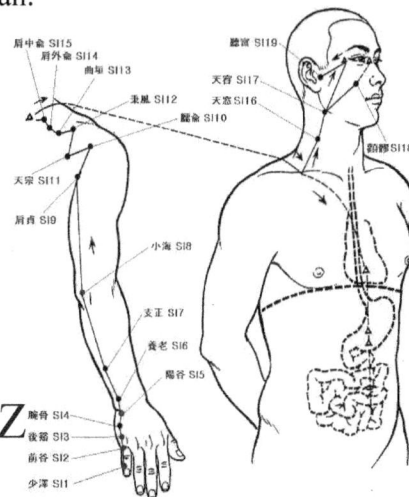

Spiritual Emotion: ASSIMILATION

Gem Essence: RUTILATED QUARTZ

Emotions: Hurting, Nervousness, Joy, Shock, Sorrow, Sadness, Internalisation, Over excited, Discouraged, Egotistical, Over confident, Conceited, Stepped On, Needy, Manipulated, Worthless

Colour the Meridian and the Acupressure Holding Point Red

Red

Triple Warmer

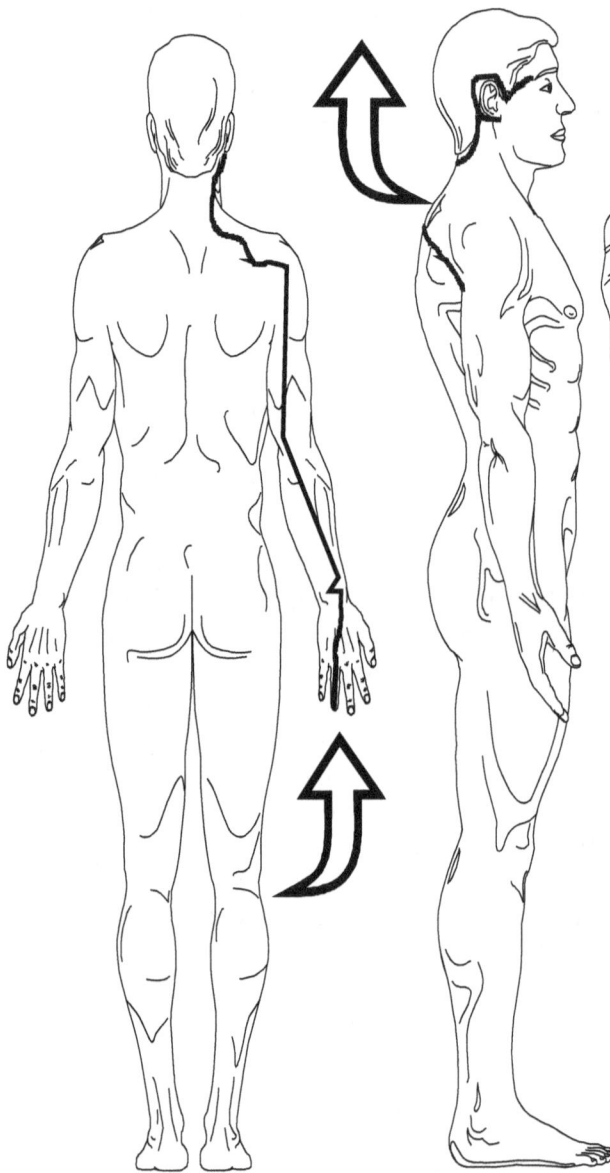

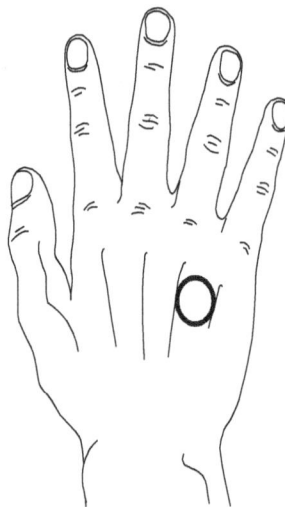

The Triple Burner Meridian beginning at the out tip of the finger, the Triple Burner Meridian proceeds over the back of the hand (1) and wrist to the forearm (2). It runs upward, passing around the outer elbow, along the lateral aspect of the upper arm (3), to reach the posterior shoulder region (4). from here, the Meridian travels over the shoulder (5) and enters into the chest underneath the breastbone. An internal branch passes from this point through the Pericardium, penetrates the diaphragm (6), and then proceeds downward (7) to unite the Upper, Middle, and Lower Burners. Another, exterior branch ascends toward the shoulder and runs internally up the neck (8). It reaches the posterior border of the ear (9) and then interiorly circles the face (10). A short branch originates behind the ear, penetrates the ear, and emerges in front of the ear (11) to reach the outer end of the eyebrow and connect to Gall Bladder Meridian.

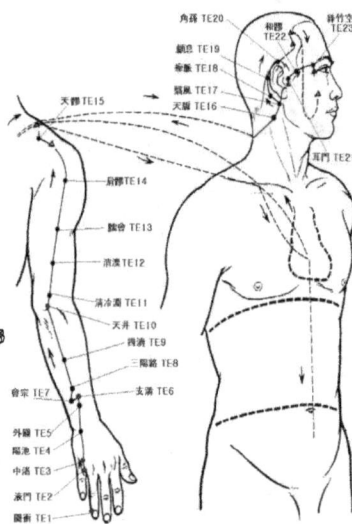

Spiritual Emotion: HARMONY

Gem Essence: GOLD, ABUNDANCE ESSENCE

Emotions: Despair, Unpleasant, Lonliness, Repulsive, Hopeless, Overexpressive, Balance, Unempathetic, Sad, Overloaded, Misunderstood, Uneasy, Insignificant, Unsatisfied, Resentful, Possessive.

Colour the Meridian and the Acupressure Holding Point Red

Red Heart

The Heart Meridian has three branches, each of which begins in the Heart (1). One branch runs downward through the diaphragm (2) to connect to the Small Intestine. A second branch runs upward from the Heart along the side of the throat (3) to meet the eye. The third branch runs across the chest from the Heart to the Lung (4), then descends and emerges in the under-arm. It passes along the midline of the inside of the upper arm (5), runs downward across the inner elbow, along the midline of the inside of the forearm (6), crosses the wrist and palm (7), and terminates at the inside tip of the little finger, where it connects with the Small Intestine Meridian.

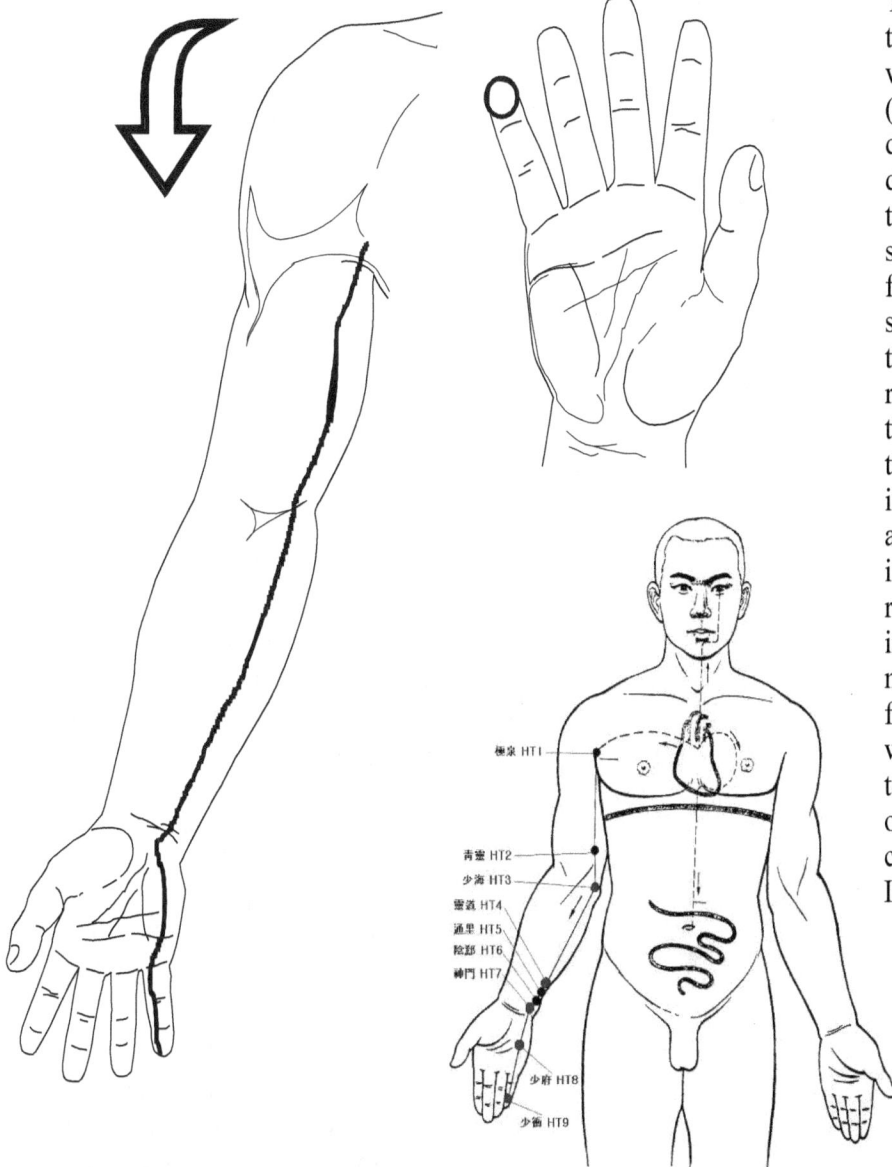

極泉 HT1
青靈 HT2
少海 HT3
靈道 HT4
通里 HT5
陰郄 HT6
神門 HT7
少府 HT8
少衝 HT9

Spiritual Emotion: UNCONDITIONAL LOVE

Emotions: Self Confidence, Infatuation, Worth, Heartbroken, Insecure, Passive, Secure, Forgetful, Hate, Apathetic, Love, Forlorn, Manipulative, Martyred, Gullible, Greedy, Ignorant. Gem Essence: Rose Quartz, Nurture Essence

Colour the Meridian and the Acupressure Holding Point Red

Red

Pericardium / Circulation Sex

Energy imbalance may be created through being unhappy with self and others.

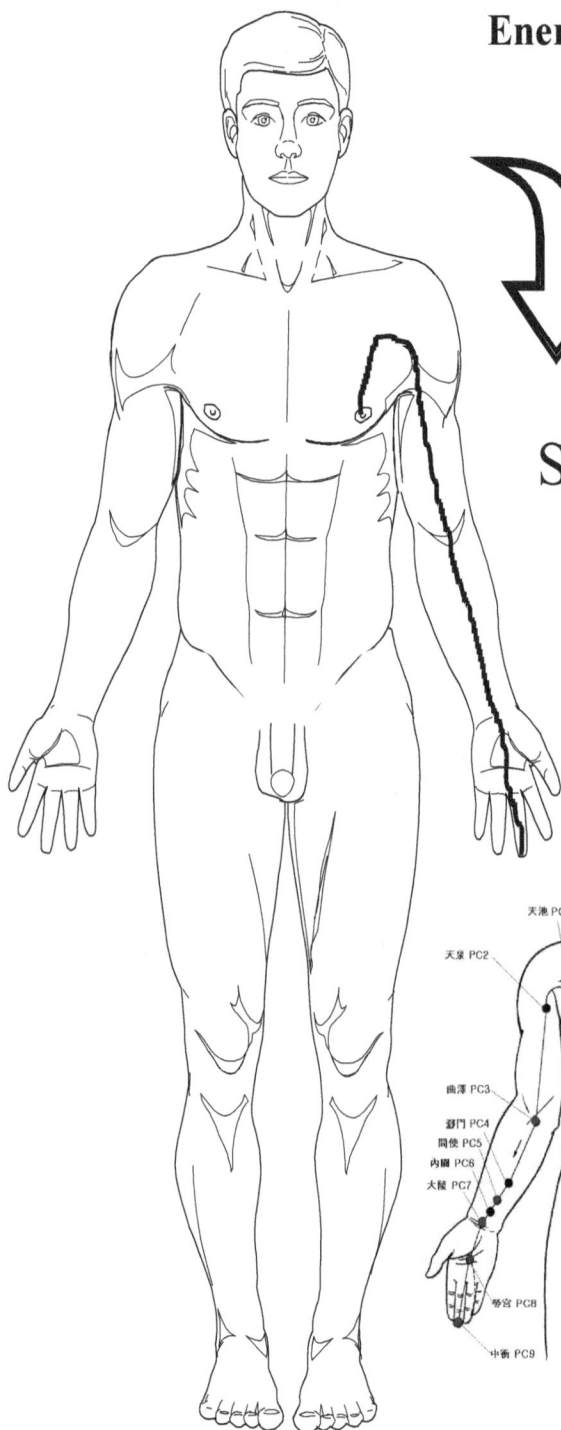

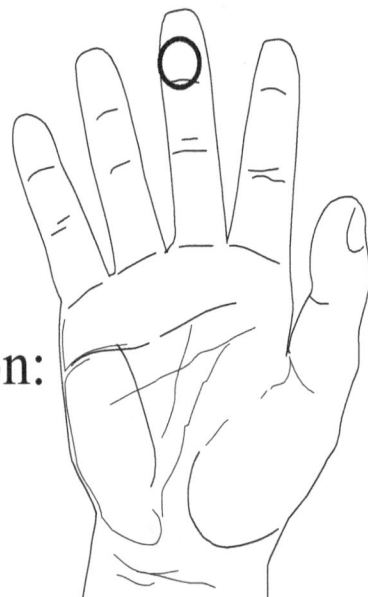

Spiritual Emotion:

BONDING

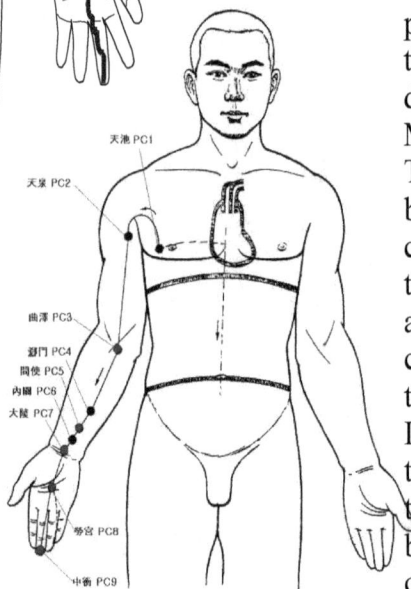

The Pericardium Meridian Beginning in the chest and in its pertaining Organ, the Pericardium (1), this Meridian descends through th diaphragm (2) to link the Upper, Middle, and Lower portions of the Triple Burner. A second internal branch of the Meridian crosses the chest (3), emerging to the surface at the area of the ribs. The Meridian then ascends around the armpit (4) and continues down the medial aspect of the upper arm (5) to the elbow crease. It runs further down the forearm (6) to the palm of the hand (7), ending at the tip of the middle finger. A short branch splits off from the palm (8) to connect with the Triple Burner Meridian at the end of the ring finger.

天池 PC1
天泉 PC2
曲澤 PC3
郄門 PC4
間使 PC5
內關 PC6
大陵 PC7
勞宮 PC8
中衝 PC9

Emotions: Hysteria, Tied Down, Stubbornness, Choiceless, Jealousy, Purposeless, Remorse, In the Dark, Incapable, Used, Indifferent, Hostile.

Gem Essence: JASPER

Color the Meridian and the Acupressure Holding Point Red

Yellow Stomach

⬇

Energy imbalance may be created through Matters of Judgement of self and others.

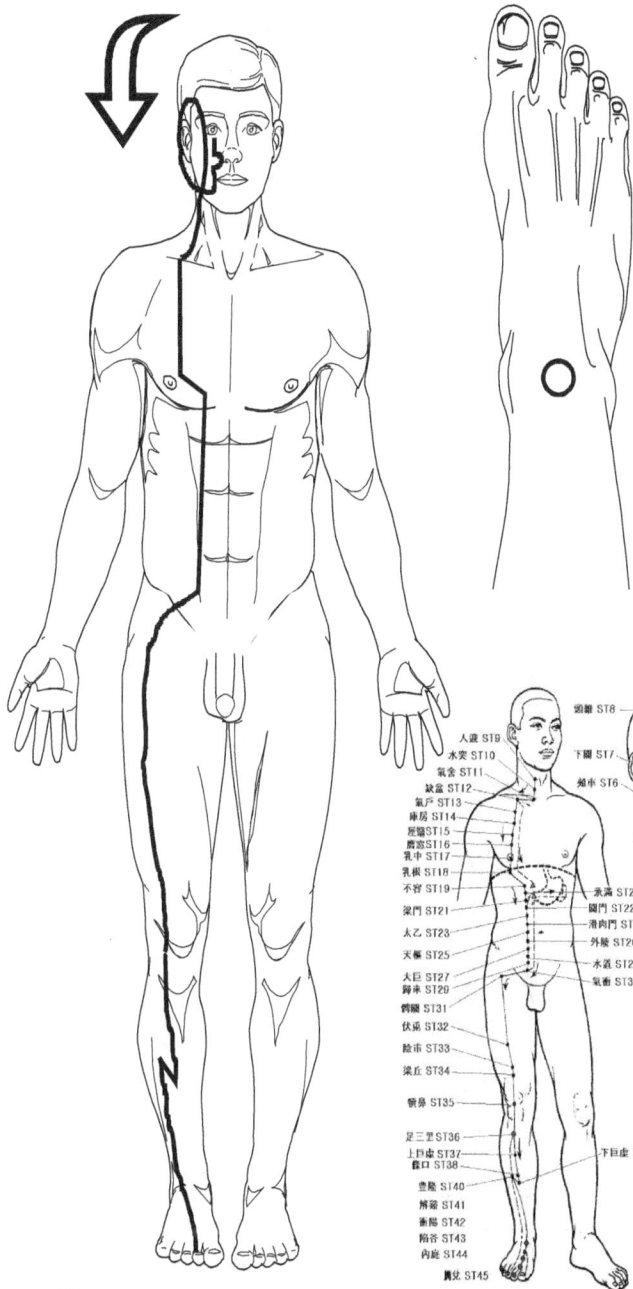

The Stomach Meridian begins, internally, where the Large Intestine Meridian terminates, next to the nose (1). It then ascends to the bridge of the nose, meeting the Bladder Meridian at the inner corner of the eye, and emerging under the eye. Descending from there, lateral to the nose, it enters the upper gum (2) and curves around the lips before passing along the side of the lower jawbone (3) and through the angle of the jaw. It then turns upward, running in front of the ear (4) to the corner of the forehead. A branch descends from the lower jaw (5), enters the body, and descends through the diaphragm. It then enters its pertaining Organ, the Stomach, and connects with the Spleen (6). Another branch leaves the lower jaw, but remains on the surface of the body as it crosses over the neck, chest (7), and abdomen (8), and terminates in the groin. Internally, the Meridian reconstitutes itself at the lower end of the stomach and descends inside the abdomen (9) to reconnect with the external branch in the groin. From this point, the Meridian runs downward over the front of the thigh (10) to the outer side of the knee (11), and continues along the center of the front of the lower leg to reach the top of the foot. It terminates at the lateral side of the tip of the second toe. A branch deviates from the Stomach Meridian just below the knee (12) and ends at the lateral side of the middle toe. A short branch also leaves from the top of the foot (13) and terminates at the medial side of the big toe to connect with the Spleen Meridian.

Gem Essence: CITRINE
Spiritual Emotion: CONTENTMENT

Emotions: Contentment, Deprivation, Disappointed, Submissive, Sympathy, Gullible, Empathy, Condescending, Disgust, Refusal to leave comfort zone, Unaccepting, Worried, Frightened, Undetermined.

Colour the Meridian and the Acupressure Holding Point Yellow

39

Yellow Spleen

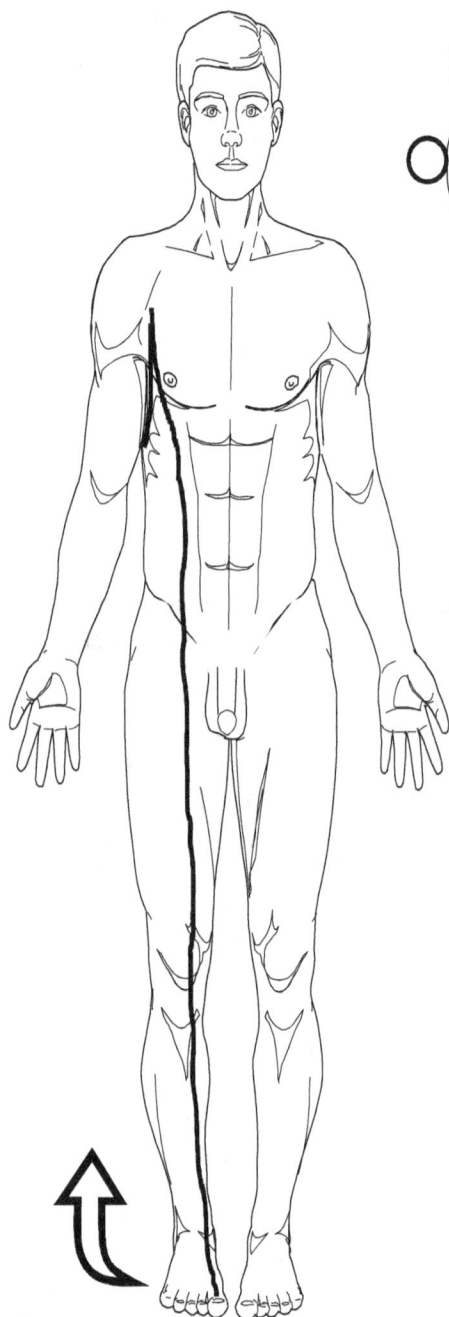

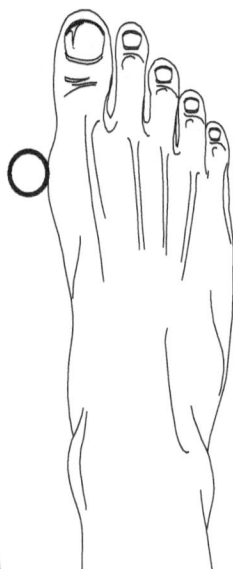

The Spleen Meridian originates at the medial side of the big toe. It then runs along the inside of the foot (1) turning in front of the inner ankle bone. From there, it ascends along the posterior surface of the lower leg (2) and the medial aspect of the knee and thigh (3) to enter the abdominal cavity (4). It runs internally to its pertaining Organ, the Spleen (5), and connects with the Stomach (6). The main Meridian continues on the surface of the abdomen, running upward to the chest (7), where it again penetrates internally to follow the throat (8) up to the root of the tongue (9), under which it spreads its Qi and Blood. An internal branch leaves the Stomach, passes upward through the diaphragm, and enters into the Heart (10), where it connects with the Heart Meridian.

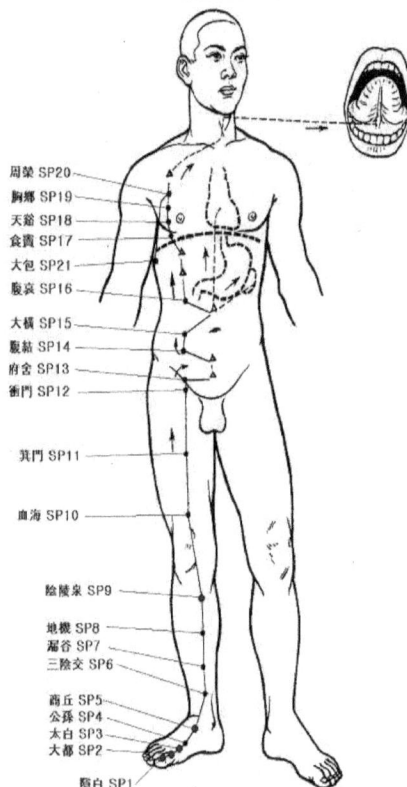

周榮 SP20
胸鄉 SP19
天谿 SP18
食竇 SP17
大包 SP21
腹哀 SP16
大橫 SP15
腹結 SP14
府舍 SP13
衝門 SP12
箕門 SP11
血海 SP10
陰陵泉 SP9
地機 SP8
漏谷 SP7
三陰交 SP6
商丘 SP5
公孫 SP4
太白 SP3
大都 SP2
隱白 SP1

Gem Essence: JADE
Spiritual Emotion: REFLECTION

Emotions: Faith in the future, Alienation, Conceited, Sympathy, Empathy, Betrayed, Useless, Envy, Foolhardy, Unhappy, Cowardly, Blaming, Disappointed, Deprived.

Colour the Meridian and the Acupressure Holding Point Yellow

White Lung

Energy imbalance may be created through Negative thinking.

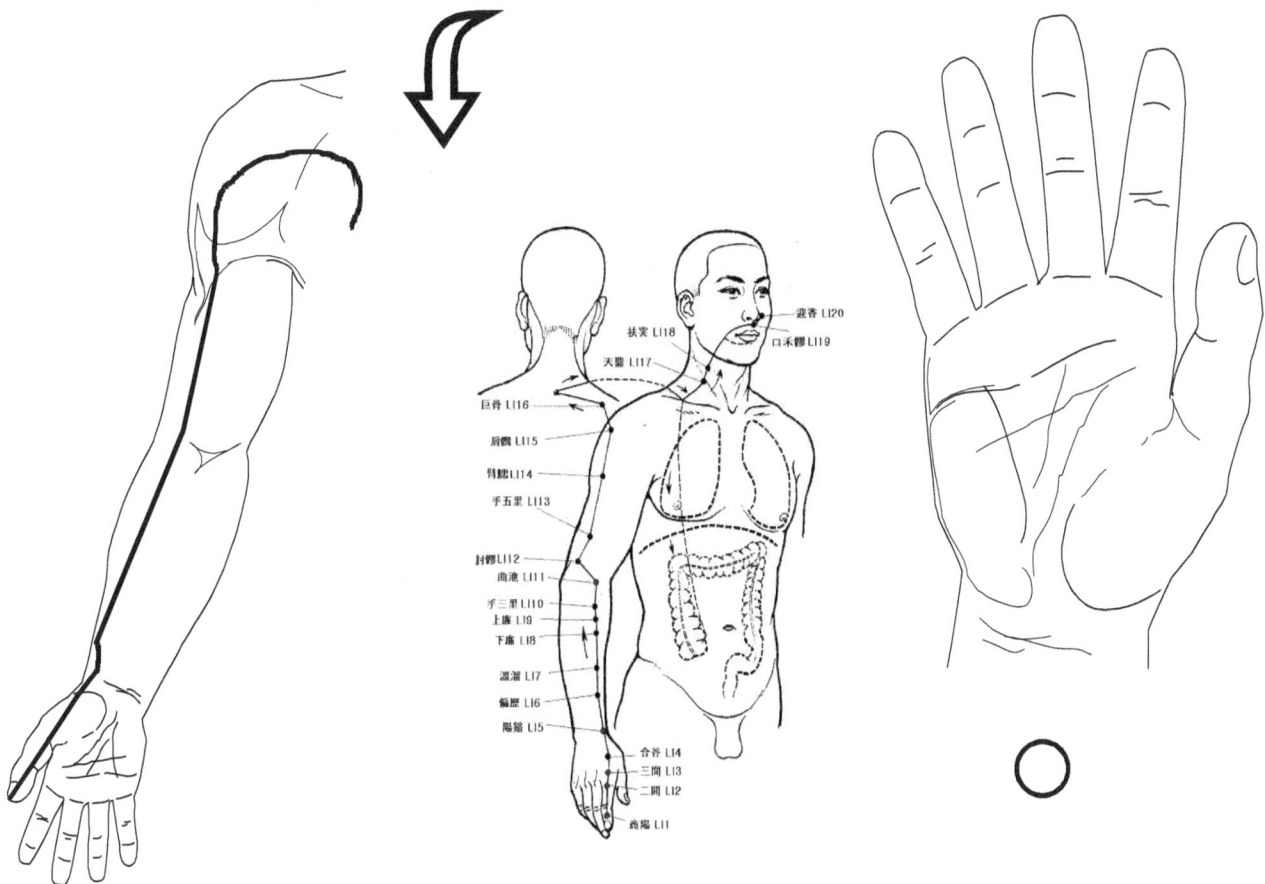

迎香 LI20
口禾髎 LI19
扶突 LI18
天鼎 LI17
巨骨 LI16
肩髃 LI15
臂臑 LI14
手五里 LI13
肘髎 LI12
曲池 LI11
手三里 LI10
上廉 LI9
下廉 LI8
温溜 LI7
偏歷 LI6
陽谿 LI5
合谷 LI4
三間 LI3
二間 LI2
商陽 LI1

The Lung Meridian originates in the middle portion of the body cavity (1) and runs downward, internally, to connect with the Large Intestine (2). Turning back, it passes upward through the diaphragm (3) to enter its pertaining Organ, the Lungs (4). From the internal zone between the Lungs and the throat (5), it emerges to the surface of the body under the clavicle. Descending, the Lung Meridian then runs along the medial aspect of the upper arm (6) to reach the elbow crease. From there, it runs along the anterior portion of the forearm (7), passes above the major artery of the wrist, and emerges at the radial side of the tip of the thumb (8). Another section of the Lung Meridian branches off just above the wrist and runs directly to the radial side of the tip of the index finger (9) to connect with the Large Intestine Meridian.

Emotions: Haughty, Suffocated, Humility, Hampered, Scorned, Bold, Disdain, Hurtful, Intolerance, Dead, Unnurtured, Destructive.

Spiritual Emotion: WORTH   Gem Essence: AZURITE

Color the Meridian and the Acupressure Holding Point Purple (White Disc)

41

White Large Intestine

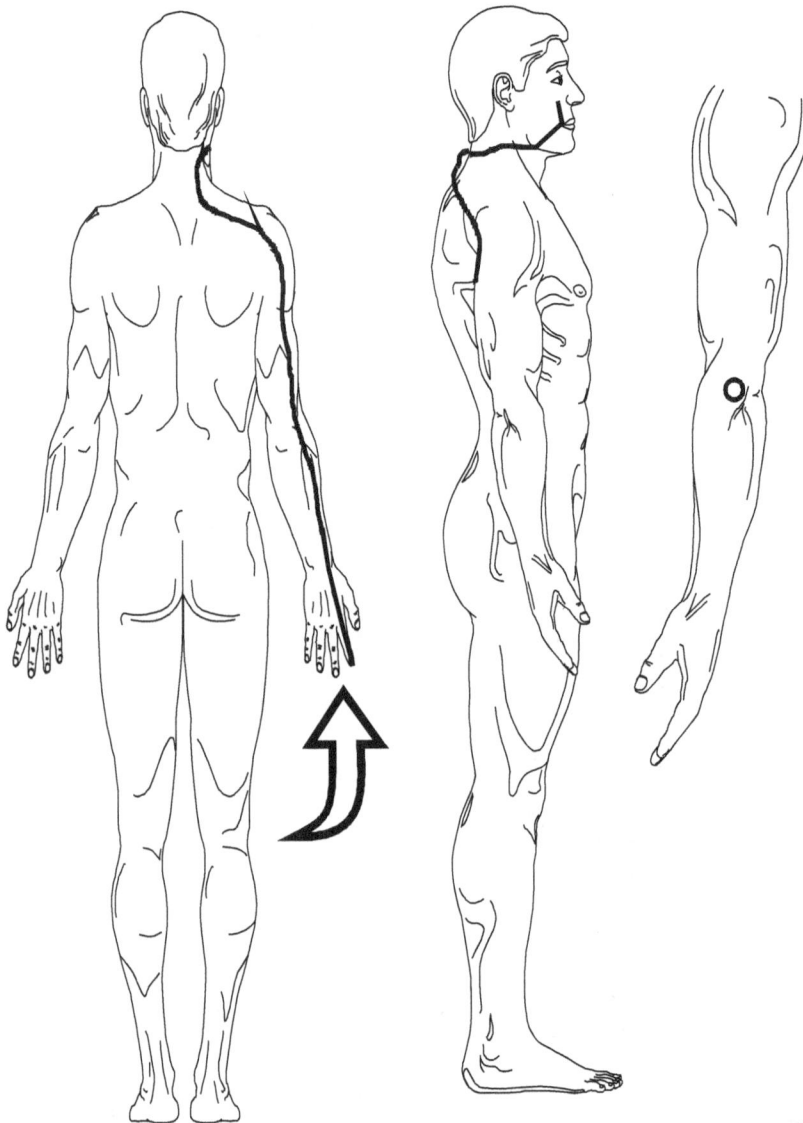

The Large Intestine Meridian begins at the tip of the index finger, and runs upward along the radial side of the index finger (1) and between the thumb and index finger. It passes through the depression between the tendons of the thumb (2) and then continues upward along the lateral aspect of the forearm to the lateral side of the elbow. From there, it ascends along the anterior border of the upper arm (3) to the highest point of the shoulder (4). On top of the shoulder, the Meridian divides into two branches (5). The first of these branches enters the body and passes through the Lung (6), diaphragm, and the Large Intestine (7), its pertaining Organ. The second of these branches ascends externally along the neck (8), passes through the cheek (9), and enters, internally, the lower teeth and gum (10). On the exterior, it continues, curving around the upper lip and crossing to the opposite side of the nose.

迎香 LI20
扶突 LI18
口禾髎 LI19
天鼎 LI17
巨骨 LI16
肩髃 LI15
臂臑 LI14
手五里 LI13
肘髎 LI12
曲池 LI11
手三里 LI10
上廉 LI9
下廉 LI8
溫溜 LI7
偏歴 LI6
陽谿 LI5
合谷 LI4
三間 LI3
二間 LI2
商陽 LI1

Spiritual Emotion:
LETTING GO

Gem Essence: AMBER

Emotions: Release, Sorrowful, Indifference, Inadequate, Apathy, Weary, Unmotivated, Vindictive, Greedy, Reclusive, Envious.

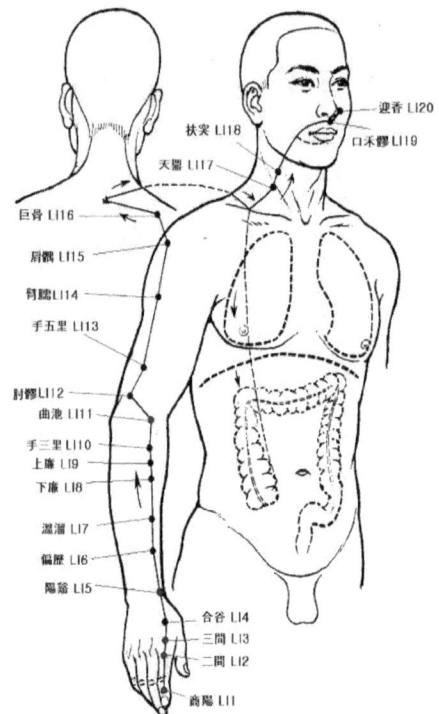

Colour the Meridian and the Acupressure Holding Point Purple (White Disc)

Blue Kidney

1.

2.

3.

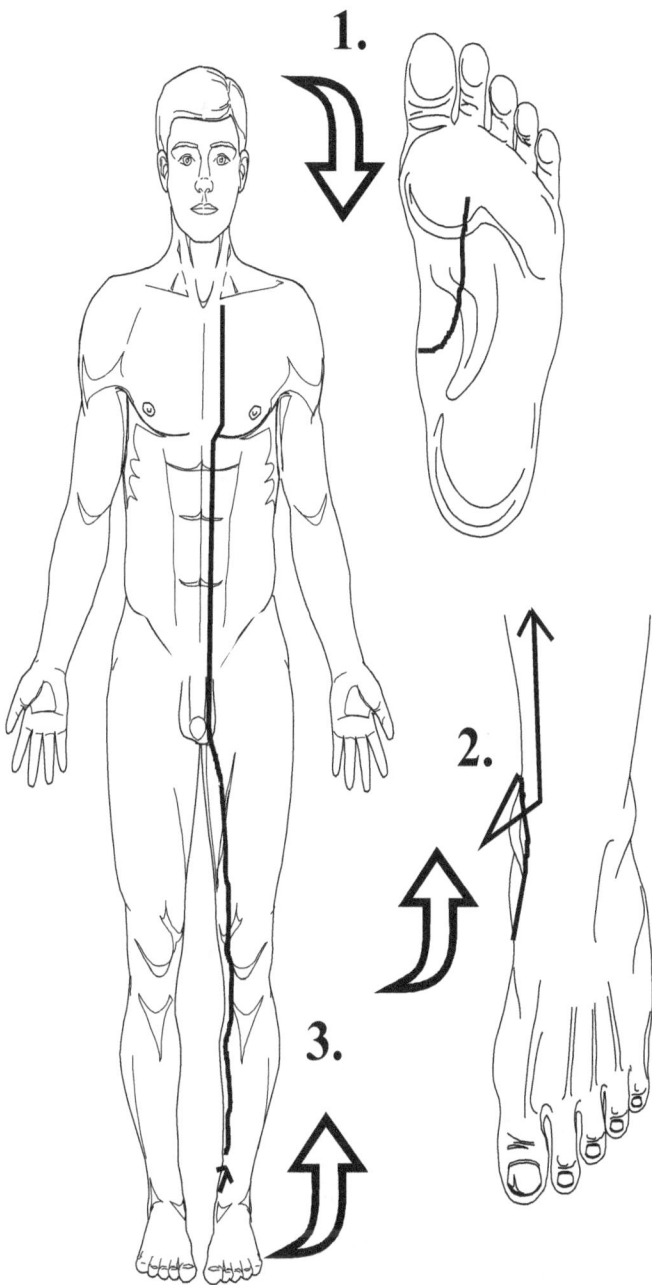

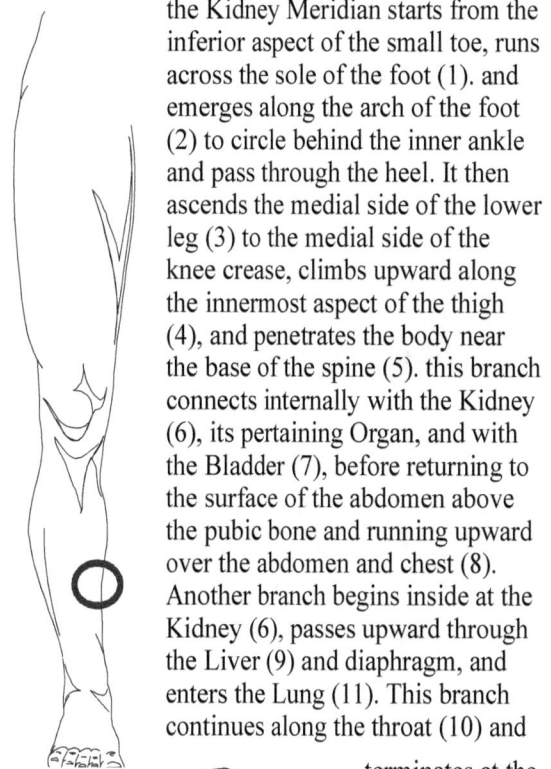

the Kidney Meridian starts from the inferior aspect of the small toe, runs across the sole of the foot (1). and emerges along the arch of the foot (2) to circle behind the inner ankle and pass through the heel. It then ascends the medial side of the lower leg (3) to the medial side of the knee crease, climbs upward along the innermost aspect of the thigh (4), and penetrates the body near the base of the spine (5). this branch connects internally with the Kidney (6), its pertaining Organ, and with the Bladder (7), before returning to the surface of the abdomen above the pubic bone and running upward over the abdomen and chest (8). Another branch begins inside at the Kidney (6), passes upward through the Liver (9) and diaphragm, and enters the Lung (11). This branch continues along the throat (10) and

terminates at the root of the tongue. A smaller branch leaves the Lung (11), joins the Heart, and flows into the chest to connect with the Pericardium Meridian.

極泉 HT1

青靈 HT2
少海 HT3
靈道 HT4
通里 HT5
陰郄 HT6
神門 HT7

少府 HT8
少衝 HT9

Spiritual Emotion: GENTLE SPIRIT
Gem Essence: SODALITE

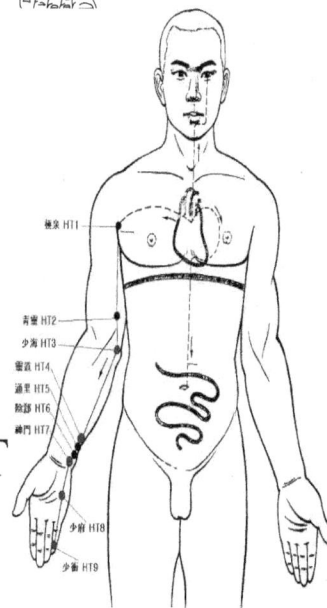

Emotions
Anxiety, Misunderstood, Blaming, Intolerant, Sexual insecurity, Creative Insecurity, Passive, Gullible, Careless, Deceitful, Self Restraint, Unloyal, Reckless, Disbelieving, Reactive, Going against intuition.

Colour the Meridian and the Acupressure Holding Point Blue

Blue

Bladder

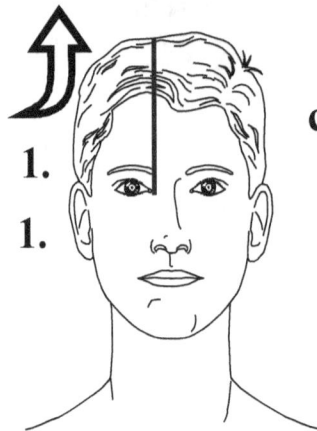

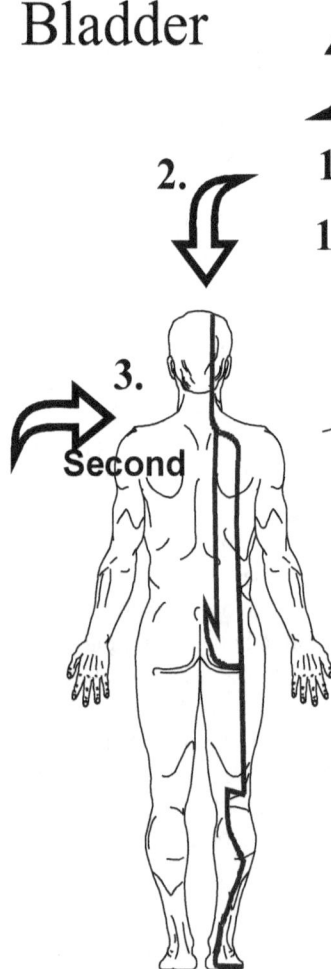

1.

2.

1.

1.

3.

Second

Energy imbalance may be created through Anxiety for self and others .

Spiritual Emotion:

INNER DIRECTION

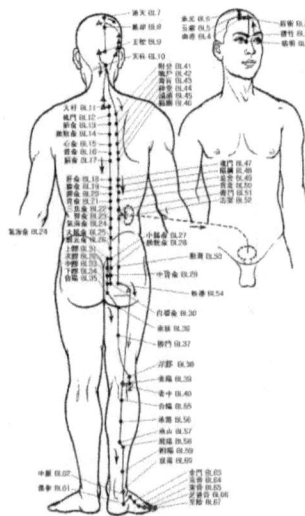

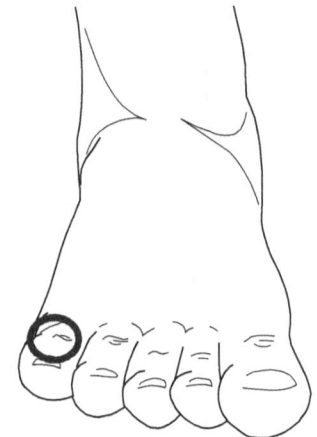

Emotions:

Fear, Anxiety, Daydreaming, Useless, Dread,

Discarded, Panic, Weary, Frustration, Weighed Down,
Sceptical, Jealous, Haughty, Purposeless, Unappreciated.

Gem Essence: AQUAMARINE

Color The Meridian and the Acupressure point Blue

The Bladder Meridian starts at the inner side of the eye and ascends across the forehead (1) to the vertex of the head. From the point, a small branch splits off and enters into the brain (2), while the main Meridian continues to descend along the back of the head (3) and bifurcates at the back of the neck (4). The inner of these two branches descends a short distance to the centre of the base of the neck (5), then descends parallel to the spine (6). A branch splits off, entering the body in the lumbar region and connecting the Kidney (7) and its pertaining Organ, the Bladder (8). The outer branch traverses the back of the shoulder (9), descends adjacent to the inner branch and the spinal cord, and crosses the buttocks (10). The two branches continue downward, descend the posterior aspect of the thigh (11), and join behind the knee. The single Meridian now continues down the back of the lower leg (12), circles behind the outer ankle, runs along the outside of the foot (13), and terminates on the lateral side of the tip of the small toe, where it connects with the Kidney Meridian

Green

Energy imbalance may be created through hurt resentment (not bitter resentment).

Gall Bladder

Spiritual Emotion:
CHOICE MAKING

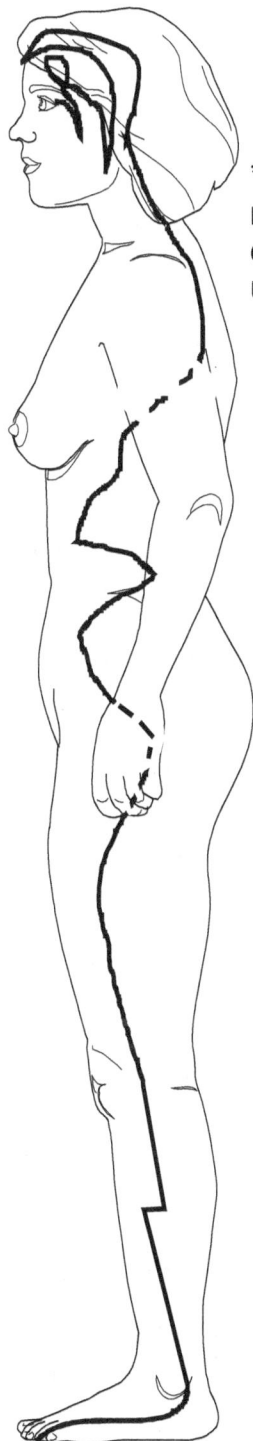

NOTE Gall Bladder meridian runs up side of body (not arm) under armpit.

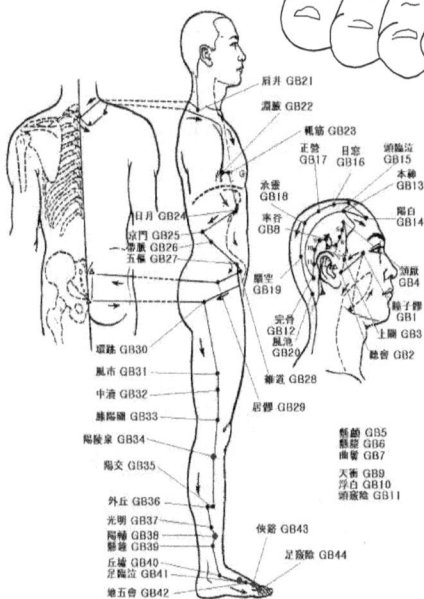

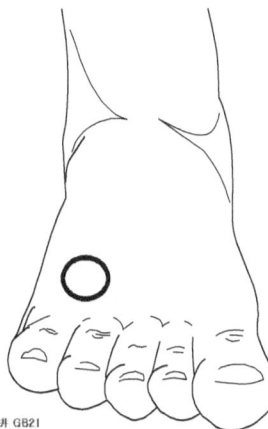

The Gall Bladder Meridian begins at the outer corner of the eye (1), where two branches arise. One branch, remaining on the surface, weaves back and forth on the lateral aspect of the head before curving behind the ear (2) to reach the top of the shoulder. It then continues downward, passing in front of the under-arm (2) and along the lateral aspect fo the rib cage (4) to reach the hip region. The second branch internally traverse the cheek (5) and proceeds internally through the neck (6) and chest (7) to reach the Liver and its pertaining Organ, the Gall Bladder (8).

Continuing downward, this branch emerges on the side of the lower abdomen, where it connects with the other branch in the hip area (9). The Meridian then descends along the lateral aspect of the thigh (10) and knee to the side of the lower leg (11) and further downward in front of the outer ankle. It crosses the top of the foot (12) and terminates at the lateral side of the tip of the fourth toe. A branch leaves the Meridian just below the ankle to cross over the foot (13) to the big toe, where it connects with the Liver Meridian.

肩井 GB21
淵腋 GB22
輒筋 GB23
正營 GB17　日窓 GB16　頭臨泣 GB15　本神 GB13
承靈 GB18　　　陽白 GB14
日月 GB24
京門 GB25　腦空 GB26　五樞 GB27　顱息 GB4
腦空 GB19　絲竹空 GB1　上關 GB3　聽會 GB2
完骨 GB12　風池 GB20
維道 GB28
居髎 GB29
懸顱 GB5　懸釐 GB6　曲鬢 GB7　天衝 GB9　浮白 GB10　頭竅陰 GB11
環跳 GB30
風市 GB31
中瀆 GB32
膝陽關 GB33
陽陵泉 GB34
陽交 GB35
外丘 GB36
光明 GB37
陽輔 GB38　懸鐘 GB39
丘墟 GB40　足臨泣 GB41
地五會 GB42
俠谿 GB43
足竅陰 GB44

Emotions: Pushed, Intolerant, Uprooted, Overconfident. Anger, Choice, Rage, Egotistical, Mean, Low self esteem, Adoration, Easily Manipulated, Sloppy, Helpless, Arrogant, Humble, Immaculate,

Gem Essence: SAPPHIRE

Colour the Meridian and the Acupressure Holding Point Green

Green

Liver

Energy imbalance may be created through Overwrought anger and bitter resentment.

Spiritual Emotion:

TRANSFORMATION

The Liver Meridian

Beginning on the top of the big toe, the Liver Meridian traverses the top of the foot (1). ascending in front of the inner ankle and along the medial aspect of the lower leg (2) and knee. It runs continuously along the medial aspect of the thigh (3) to the pubic region, where it encircles the external genitalia (4) before entering the lower abdomen. It ascends internally (5), connects with its pertaining Organ, the Liver (6), and with the Gall Bladder, and scatter s underneath the ribs (7) before pouring into the Lungs (8), where it connects with the Lung Meridian (Fig. 3). The entire cycle of the Meridian system begins anew here. Reconstituting

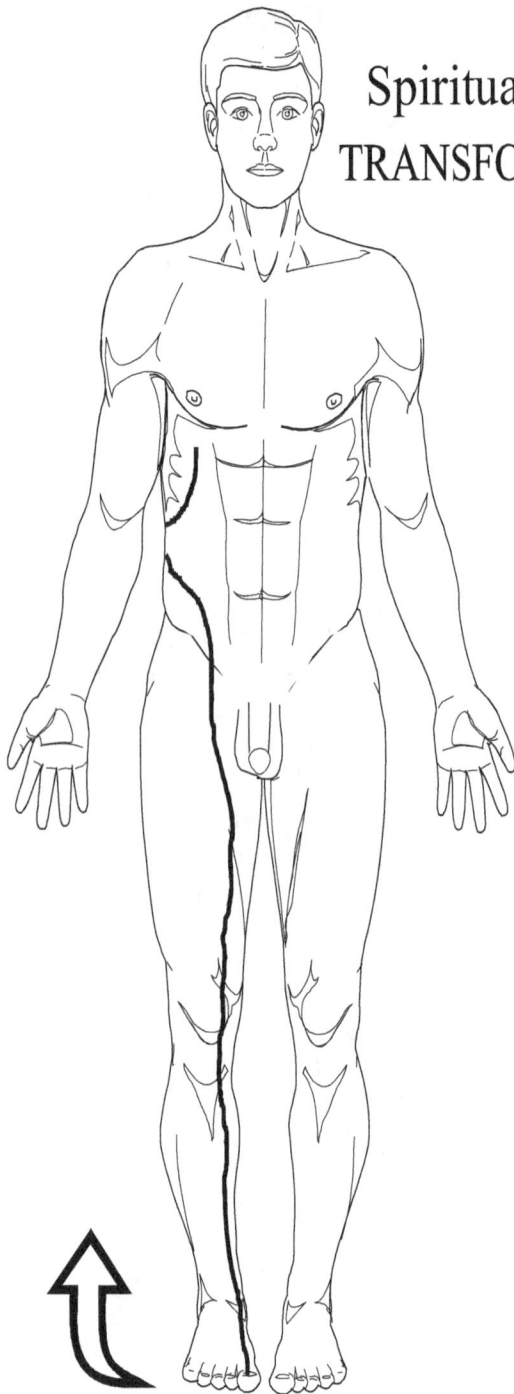

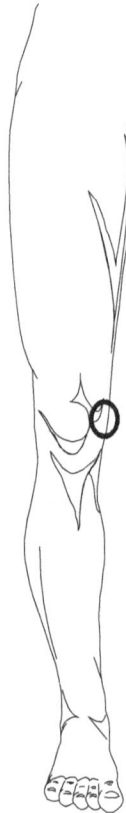

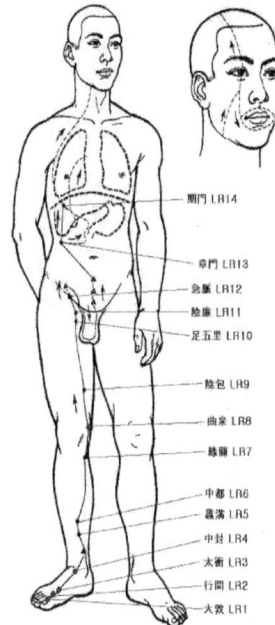

itself, the Meridian follows the trachea upward to the throat (9) and connects with the eyes (10). Two branches leave the eye area: One descends across the cheek to encircle the inner surface of the lips (11); a second branch ascends across the forehead (12) to reach the vertex of the head.

期門 LR14
章門 LR13
急脈 LR12
陰廉 LR11
足五里 LR10
陰包 LR9
曲泉 LR8
膝關 LR7
中都 LR6
蠡溝 LR5
中封 LR4
太衝 LR3
行間 LR2
大敦 LR1

Gem Essence: PERIDOT

Emotions: Rage, Irritability, Distressed, Morbid, Daring, Resentment, Annoyed, Ruthless, Responsibility, Boisterous, Transformation, Unhappiness, Unprotected, Vindicated, Unreceptive, Unadaptable, Unimportant, Incomplete.

Colour the Meridian and the Acupressure Holding Point Green

Meridian Checking Points

Please note: Meridian checking points are always located on both sides of the body (except for Central & Governing)

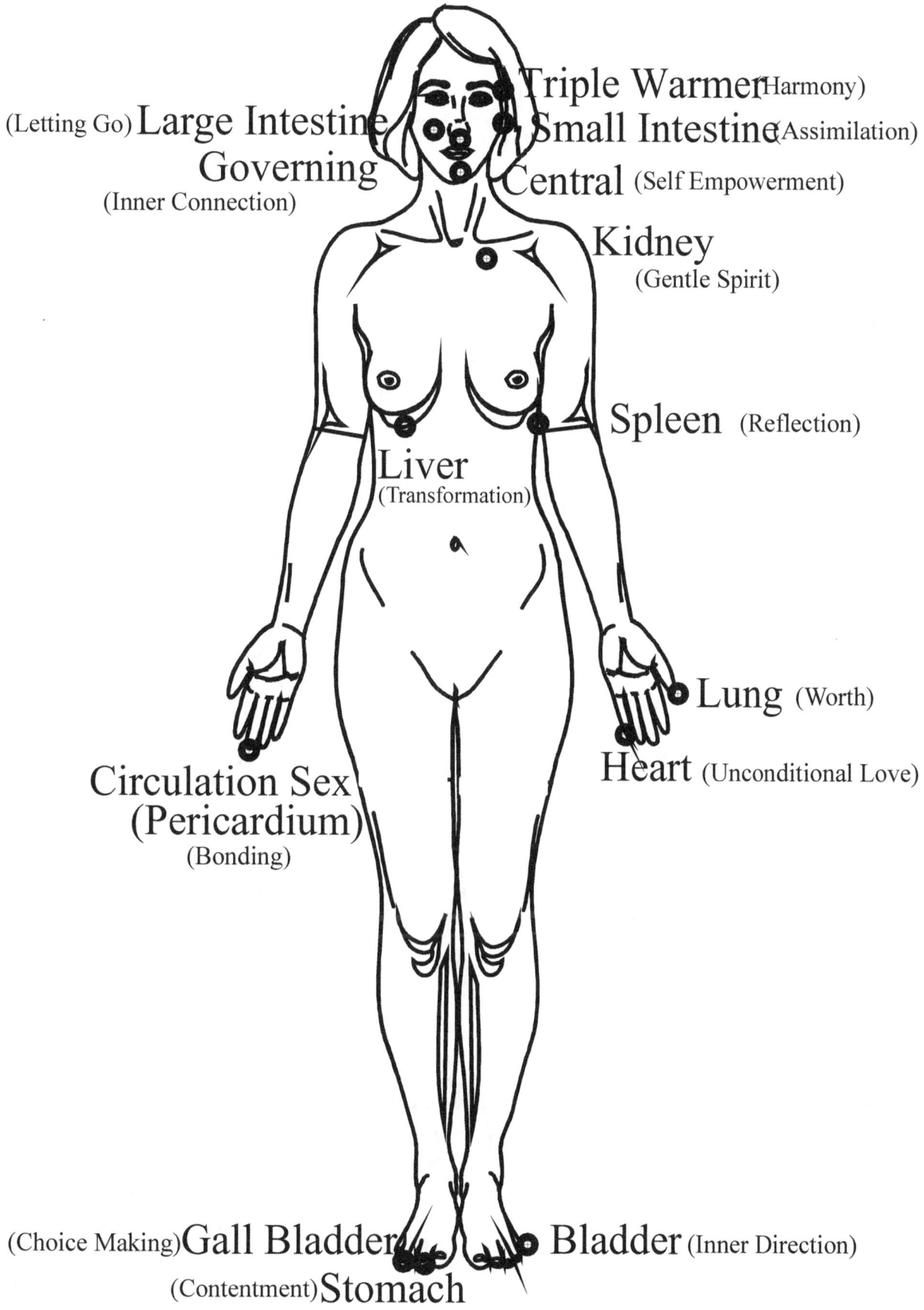

(Letting Go) Large Intestine

Triple Warmer (Harmony)

Small Intestine (Assimilation)

Governing
(Inner Connection)

Central (Self Empowerment)

Kidney
(Gentle Spirit)

Spleen (Reflection)

Liver
(Transformation)

Lung (Worth)

Circulation Sex
(Pericardium)
(Bonding)

Heart (Unconditional Love)

(Choice Making) Gall Bladder

Bladder (Inner Direction)

(Contentment) Stomach

47

Checking Points For Acupressure Holding Points

Please note: Acupressure checking points are always located on both sides of the body

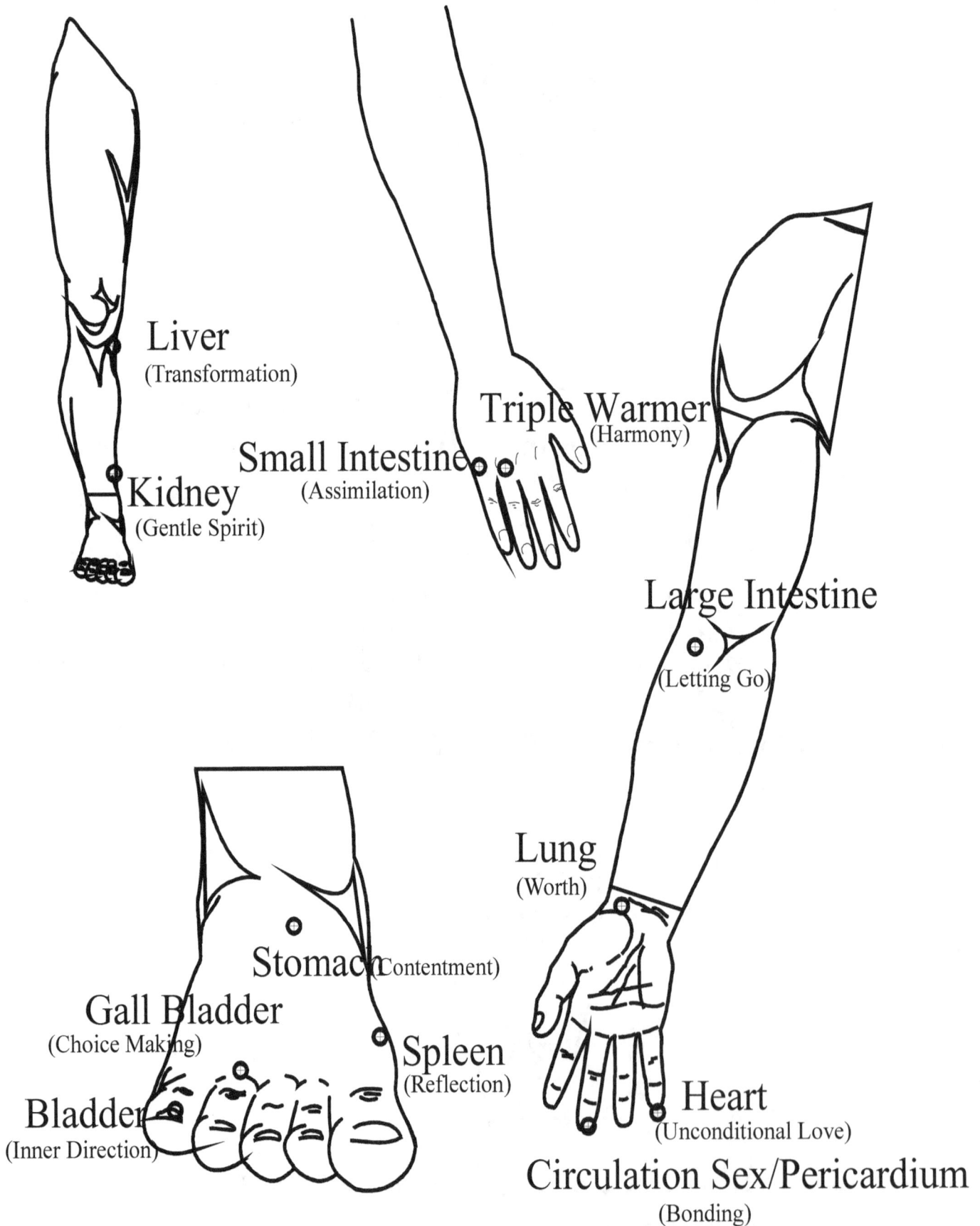

Liver
(Transformation)

Triple Warmer
(Harmony)

Small Intestine
(Assimilation)

Kidney
(Gentle Spirit)

Large Intestine

(Letting Go)

Lung
(Worth)

Stomach (Contentment)

Gall Bladder
(Choice Making)

Spleen
(Reflection)

Bladder
(Inner Direction)

Heart
(Unconditional Love)

Circulation Sex/Pericardium
(Bonding)

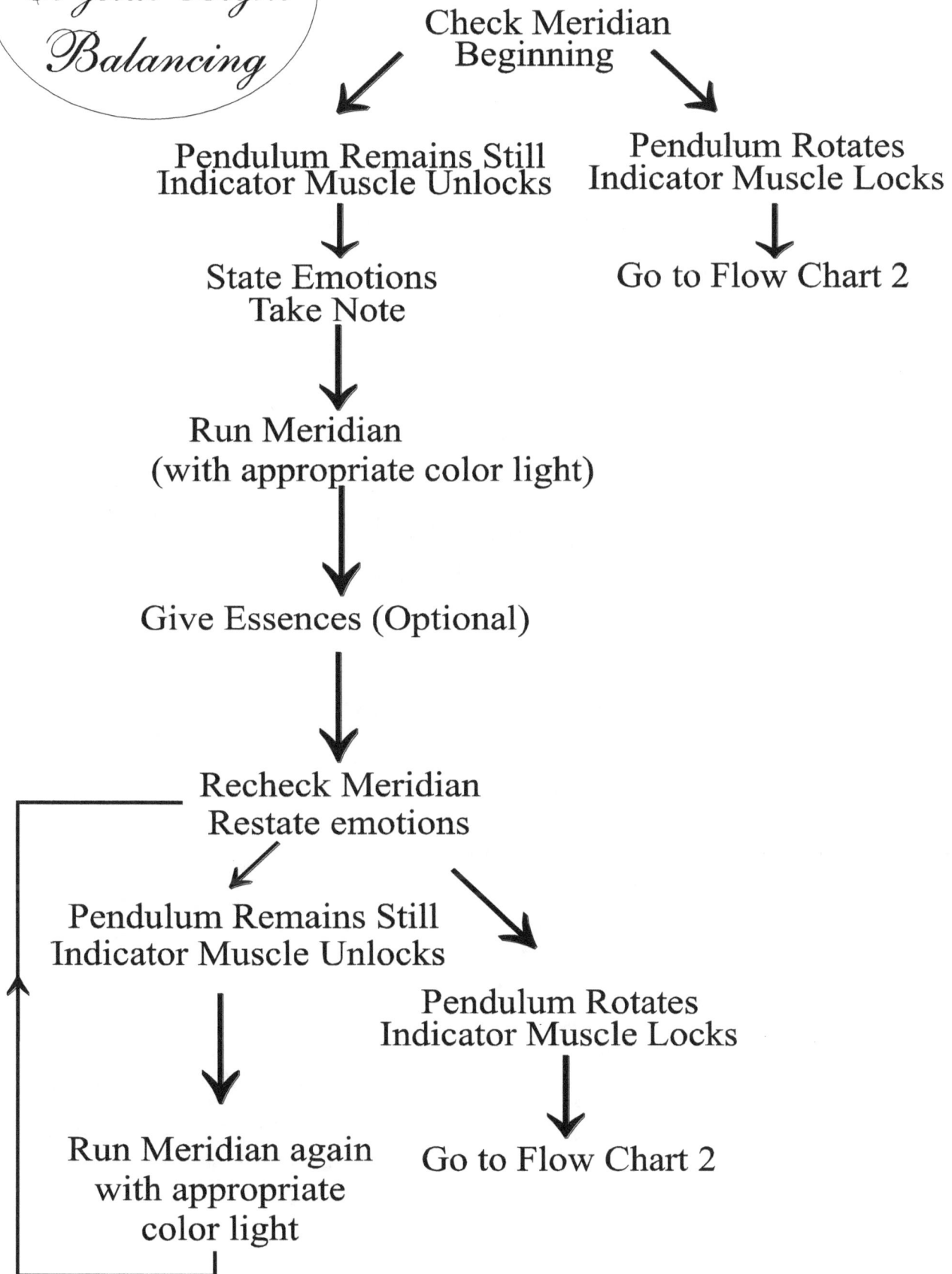

Renascent Crystal Light Balancing

Flow Chart 1

Check Meridian
Beginning

Pendulum Remains Still
Indicator Muscle Unlocks

Pendulum Rotates
Indicator Muscle Locks

State Emotions
Take Note

Go to Flow Chart 2

Run Meridian
(with appropriate color light)

Give Essences (Optional)

Recheck Meridian
Restate emotions

Pendulum Remains Still
Indicator Muscle Unlocks

Pendulum Rotates
Indicator Muscle Locks

Run Meridian again
with appropriate
color light

Go to Flow Chart 2

Flow Chart 2

Renascent Crystal Light Balancing

Check Acupressure Holding Point

Pendulum Remains Still
Indicator Muscle Unlocks

Pendulum Rotates
Indicator Muscle Locks

State Emotions
Take Note

Hold appropriate color light
on point: 30 - 60 Seconds

Give Essences (Optional)

14 Meridians Checked ?

Recheck Point
Restate emotions

Pendulum Remains Still
Indicator Muscle Unlocks

Hold Light for
longer time

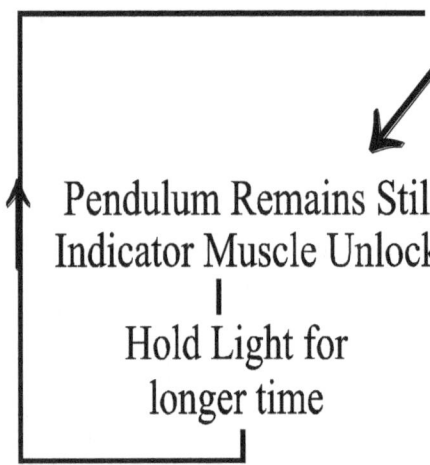

Pendulum Rotates
Indicator Muscle Locks

No

Yes

Go to next
Meridian
& Flow Chart 1

Process
Complete

Previous Topics Discussed

As you have read through this book, there has been reference to topics that you may not be familiar with. I will briefly explain them here.

CAN I USE ANY GEM ESSENCES, INCLUDING THOSE I MAKE MYSELF ?

I do not recommend any Gem Essences other than the Renascent variety. I know that sounds like a sales pitch as I am directly involved with Renascent. However, even if I wasn't this would still be my response. There are many products that Renascent supply that we will happily share how to make yourself if you desire to do so, whilst still supplying them for those who wish to purchase their products. Essences are in many cases undermined as people CAN make them very easily. However, the essences that have been made in a very simple manner in my experience have limited or no healing benefits.

Usually this is as a result or lack of information or dedication to the quality of the essences. *The following is an extract from the Gem Essence Workbook*

Gem essences are prepared in many ways similar to flower essences, however with more knowledge now available on other factors such as electromagnetic radiation and pollution we are able to offer more in depth manners of preparation which in turn makes the essences even more beneficial.

Many people prepare their gem essence by taking a glass bowl outside, filling it with distilled water, placing their gem in it and leaving it there in the sun for two hours.

This method will work <u>to a very limited degree</u>, yet there are some major concerns here that this is not taking into consideration. In pursuit for particularly effective and potentised essences, I believe these factors are crucial.

Firstly there is the electromagnetic fields which run through the earth which may be energy polluted and in turn may pass through into the water and may contaminate the essence, in the sense of producing a debilitating stress response to the subtle bodies. The very area vibrational medicine seeks to heal. Then there is the factor of aeroplanes or jets passing overhead which emit not only electromagnetic pollution, but also electromagnetic radiation from their radar equipment. Any of these fields when tested in muscle testing, the body cannot hold a lock to, ie - the body cannot maintain its strength. Should these fields be present when the essence is being made then it will be locked into the water and retain a subatomic message of these fields. When used for healing, any such essence cannot have a potentised healing effect on the body.

There are also bacteria concerns to look at through leaving an uncovered bowl of water in the sun outside for some time. These factors may seem particularly subtle, however I am sure I have no need to remind you that it is this area of subtlety we are working in.

This chapter is not to teach you how to create your own Gem Essences, for without the correct equipment, Geological Knowledge and background you would probably, at the very least, make a weak and inefficient essence and at the worst could make a deadly solution.

In so many areas of my life I am tempted to step in and make something myself to cut costs and have the thrill of discovery, however much life experience has taught me that unless my life is dedicated to focus solely on that area then I am always better off to leave it to those people who are. I also see it as supporting the energies of those people who have spent years of their lives researching and creating a potentised wonderful product for me to use.

I am constantly coming across situations where people have decided to create a product purely to make money as opposed to carrying a passion for it in their heart. This is not to say there is anything wrong with people making money, however if that money is created from a product or a service that they love and hold a dear passion for, then that is what I feel it is all about. I purchase a beautiful range of skin care I love to use, it is rather costly and at one point in my life I could not justify the expense and decided to make my own. After much purchasing of equipment and ingredients I set about and created some moisturisers, however after using them for a couple of months I began to notice that my skin did not seem to have the special glow it used to. It felt a little "tired" and pale, realising I could not afford to spend the necessary time researching skin care at this point in my life (and I believe that in any area of specialty a minimum of 5-20 years study is necessary, possibly even a lifetime) I decided that I would go back to purchasing the skin care from the company again. My skin regained its glow and healthy appearance almost overnight and I said a silent thank you to the people who had invested so much of their lives and passions in creating this range for me to use. I believe the area of skin care is simply an example of any area of expertise for a product we wish to use and this understanding can be carried through in almost any product or area of our lives. If we want a job done well, then we call in the professionals.

I received a phone call from a lady some time ago, requesting that I make her an essence from a particular item (in this case it was a Pearl).

I explained that we do not make Pearl essence and asked why it was so important that she had this particular essence. It seems that she had been to a practitioner who had told her that this was what she needed to get made. I explained that we only create 40 essences (although 1 extra - Chrysoprase, has recently been added for the Blessing Oil) as these are all we find necessary for all concerns. They are what we call the "umbrella essences" meaning that all other gems and crystals healing properties will be covered by one or more of these 40 and are therefore not necessary in essence form.

Delving a little deeper, I asked for the circumstances and the emotional states that led to her needing the Pearl essence, all of the states she described would be assisted by the use of a blend of Sugilite and Moonstone essence. I suggested they could be diluted together and mailed to her if she did not have the two stock essences. However, not satisfied with this purely because a practitioner had told her that is what she needed, she continued on with her desire to obtain Pearl essence. When I again informed her it was not a standard essence we supplied, she became very agitated and started raising her voice and asking what was wrong with this company and why wouldn't we simply make it for her.

Explaining again that we felt it was already covered and therefore unnecessary, she asked if she brought us a Pearl would we consider making a batch of that essence for her. Of course, this is possible, however on realising that with equipment costs, purification and the myriad of aspects that go into creating an essence the minimum quantity available would be 4 litres at a cost of approximately $15000 (not charging for equipment already on site) she quietened down considerably. I explained that with any process that is intensive, these sort of set up costs are incurred. If I was to take her Pearl and place it in a bowl of water, in my back yard, for a few hours or even days, I could probably make her essence for about $10 - $20. Yet as the only essences I will use are dedicated to excellence, this is not something I could possibly consider to do.

An awakening dawned over her and she realised what it was I was saying to her. If this was the way she wanted to obtain Pearl essence, she could do it herself, yet if she wanted a potentised healing, chances are it would not occur through this so called essence once it was completed.

Some time back I heard of a lady who will make Gem Essences in this manner for anyone who bring her their gems. I called this lady and told her I had a piece of Cinnabar and wondered if she would make an essence of it if I brought it to her. She eagerly decided she would and it would cost me under $20 for it. Inquiring how the essence would be made, she explained she would place the stone in a bowl of water outside for some hours or days, then remove the stone and bottle the remaining water with brandy for me. I asked her if I could drink it if I chose to and she explained that they do prefer external application, however it would be perfectly safe if anyone drank this liquid. At this point I expressed that her limited Geological knowledge was quite frightening and made the suggestion that it would be a good idea for her to go and dedicate 5 - 10 years of her life studying geology or a mineralogical course to gain some awareness. Taken aback and puzzled she asked why I would suggest such a thing. I explained that she was obviously unaware that Cinnabar had a water soluble Arsenic concentration and any such stone placed in water for a period of days would naturally leech this arsenic into the water and the water would become a toxic liquid. Taken internally, depending on its concentration, at the very least would make the patient quite ill, at the worst, kill them.

I was met with silence for quite some time as this was mulled over, followed by anger and resentment at being tricked. I explained that my object was not to "trick" anyone, yet as a health practitioner it is important that providing such a service as selling essences to therapists needs a dedicated heart and possibly some further studies. She thanked me for my input and went on her way, I have noticed that the essences from this company now have printed on them "for external use only" although I do not believe the method of creating the stock essences has been amended.

At a show I attended, a gem essence manufacturer delighted in showing me their new acquisition, a large piece of Smoky Quartz, they had used to make their last batch of Smoky Quartz essence. Unfortunately, the piece in their hands was in fact clear quartz, heat treated to change the appearance into that of Smoky Quartz. Again with a geological lack of knowledge this was not detected. At the same show I came across some vibrantly colored bottles, labeled as Gem Essences. As I picked them up I noticed they rattled. On closer inspection, I found that they were simply small bottles of water with a tiny gem placed in each one - someone's idea of cashing in I guess and a method of sales I find sadly lacking in integrity.

With Gem Essences, you are looking at a product that holds the ability to release deep seated emotions, rebalance the psyche and heal the body. In anybody's understanding, this makes it an important area. We are not talking about a pleasant smelling room freshener from the supermarket, we are talking about a product to realign your very being. For me personally (and I believe anyone else also) only the purest, most potentised and effective essence should be considered. The Renascent Gem Essences guarantee this promise.

Reprinted with permission from the Gem Essence Workbook.

The gem essence course is available on correspondence (certified) and we aim to have the instructor training correspondence course completed by 2003 should you wish to become an accredited Gem Essence Instructor.

Stellar Essences

The Stellar Essences are a relatively new vibrational medicine. They were originally completed in 1996. In some ways these are a different form of essence as they are not created from anything physically accessible to us eg - a rock or a flower and whilst they have very little to do with gems and crystals if you are interested in vibrational healing they are a very worthwhile healing tool that you may be interested in. They are a form of healing where energies of astrological and cosmological influence have been harnessed in a usable form. I personally use the Stellar Essences along with the Gem Essences and the Bach Flower remedies in the College Clinic and I have generally found that to be the majority of all essences that I test up to use for clients. If you would like more information on the Stellar essences, please request a brochure or look on www.renascentcollege.com The complete STELLAR ESSENCES course is now available on correspondence & is accredited, certified & recognised. It is a mind boggling, fascinating course which we highly recommend.

Flower, Shell & Other Essences

As mentioned, I only use the Renascent Gem Essences and the Bach Flower Essences, however, there are many other varieties of flower essences, shell essences and various vibrational medicine. My suggestion is to begin with the Renascent Gem Essences & Stellar essences and then if you have a love for vibrational healing - branch out and discover what works best for you.

Ch'i Energy Products

A wonderful range of products are available for harmonisation of energetic electromagnetic stress for personal use, mobile phones, animals, children, the house and for polarisation of water. My husband & I met when we were working as distributors for an EMF protection product known as 'purple plates'. Originally we loved these products, yet over time we both individually came to the decision not to distribute these any longer around 1994 as we felt they were not doing what they promised to. 2 years after this time, the Ch'i Energy products were presented to me and I have had such wonderful success with them, that at present they are the only products I recommend in this area.

There are several other products I know of that I feel also provide benefit in these energies, however in most cases they are so expensive they are out of reach of many people. The Ch'i Energy products I feel, are effective, reasonably priced (A once off purchase and do not need to be cleansed, recharged or re tuned) and attractive.

Clearing

ELECTROMAGNETIC FIELDS: If you wish to clear electromagnetic stresses from your crystals and gems all you need to do is hold the gem, vigorously shake the crystal (to dislodge the fields), then blow onto it (automatically using the prana of your breath to cleanse it) turn your crystal over and blow on the other side. This will clear the stored EMF's from your crystal yet will not remove other peoples vibrations, the same as cleansing will remove other peoples energies but will not remove EMF's. Both are necessary to cleanse to harmonise your gem. (the Awaken Your Energies book has full instructions on techniques for cleansing other peoples energies from gems & crystals)
After this procedure the crystal is clear as long as you do not go near any EMF, a seemingly impossible task in modern life. So, perform this exercise every night to keep your jewellery and gems clear. Your other alternative is to clear your gem and then keep it near a Ch'i Energy Disc (or wear one), which seems to prevent the energies imprinting back on your gem.
You may elect to put a House disc on the premises to harmonise the EMF's of the building.
Alternatively to clear human AND EMF's from your gems and crystals if you have a practitioner Ch'i Energy Disc you may choose to simply rest your gem on it for a few minutes (or wave it over). You will find your gem is cleansed, cleared and ready to assist in healing once more. I tend to use the Ch'i Energy products quite a lot as they are so easy, simple and it doesn't matter whether I am 'positively charged' with energy or a 'bit low', they will do the work for me.
You can also use the practitioners disc to cleanse energies from your massage table in between clients, heal energy disruptions & accelerate healing energies. *Complimentary brochures are available from Renascent College.*

Feng Shui

Is the art of harmonising energies within an environment.

Together with Geomancy – which encompasses the harmonising of earth / land energies you have a complete picture for environmental solutions. Many times you may find that you correct concerns with your clients and send them home only to have them return a short times later with the exact same concern. You correct it again, ensuring you access the emotions underlying the concern, yet again the next time they return the same concerns exist. If this is taking place, you may need to enlist the assistance of an experienced Feng Shui & Geomancy consultant.

Lately there has been a wide awakening into this topic and many people believe it is simply a technical art. Deeper Feng Shui was only ever passed down from master to student and encompassed a wide range of spiritual and personal developmental practices to raise the Ch'i of the practitioner. Done correctly, it changes energies, improves wealth, relationships and put definite harmony into an environment.

Renascent offer fully certified and accredited correspondence courses in Feng Shui & Geomancy & can recommend skilled practitioners to awaken and correct the Qi of your / your clients environment.

Feng Shui & Geomancy Consultations

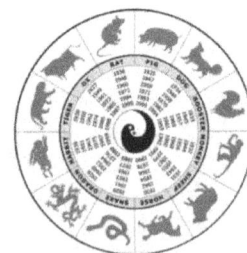

Feng Shui & Geomancy private home and business consultations. Have a trained professional give advice and recommendations for success on your environment. It is touted as the unseen advantage for any business or person. Consultations can be done in person, or if sent with house plans, photos and detailed descriptions can be completed by distance. Please contact The International College of Intuitive Sciences / Renascent College for fees or for a consultant near you.

The CLB course is a wonderful modality of healing & I'm sure you'll love it, however you will need a CLB torch to utilise this modality. Did you know that there is a CLB torch, a CLB workbook, correspondence course and set of 20 gem essences. It saves some money if you purchase them together. Postage would not increase greatly for more in the one order. The torch is now available in beautiful wooden boxes.

The CLB courses all include the eBook CLB manual. However, the manual can be purchased separately.

Renascent Crystal Light Balancing Torch

Complete in a sturdy carry case, with: Torch (batteries, clip & spare globe) Halogen globes, Quartz Crystal tip and 7 color discs. 4 for the Renascent Crystal Light Balancing & an extra 3 (no additional charge) for Chakric work. The color discs are a particular shade that produces balance in the energy systems.

ABOUT THE TORCH A stunning new healing modality tool, specially designed torches of the highest quality, specifically made with integrity for use by natural therapists. The crystal tip is made of natural, uncut and unpolished Australian Quartz crystal. Hand selected for their energies and ease of refraction. The globe is halogen to produce perfect white light thus ensuring your colors are not distorted for effective healing.

HOW TO USE THE TORCH By placing the appropriate color disc in the torch and either running this color along the appropriate meridian or holding it over the appropriate Acupressure Holding Points. Energy will be assisted to flow through these areas and balance will be achieved. Kinesiologists may muscle test which points are out of balance to determine where the torch is needed. By utilising CLB gem essences & negative & positive emotions associated with each meridian, add depth and strength to your balance.

Renascent Crystal Light Balancing Advanced Colour Discs

A lovely set of 6 additional colour discs to produce advanced colour healing as listed a little further on.

Renascent Crystal Light Balancing Workbook

The workbook given as part of the Crystal Light Balancing course.
Chinese five elements, energy flow to organs, imbalanced emotional states. Crystal pendulums, Seasonal changes, healing, Circular polarisation of light, cleansing energy blocks, Color Therapy & spiral Energy Flows, Meridian & Acupressure Holding Points, Qi or Chi flow within the body, Gem Essences, Kinesiology & Pendulum corrections pages as well as step by step instructions to inform, entice and assist you. To enhance treatments of natural therapists & for those with no prior experience.

Renascent Crystal Light Balancing Gem Essences

The gem essence kit designed to work with the Crystal Light Balancing manual (Book) & seminar, however it may be used alone. The kit contains 20 pure stock strength (not dilutions) gem essences especially chosen to rebalance emotions that cause meridian imbalance. All essences and their appropriate use for each meridian are listed in the Renascent Crystal Light Balancing Workbook. A beautiful method of healing & bringing back clarity and a feeling of greater empowerment.

Crystal Light Balancing Correspondence Course

Color therapy, Kinesiology, Pendulums, Chinese 5 elements, deep emotional balancing. An exciting powerful & deeply aligning natural therapy correction. For beginners & practitioners alike
Course contains: Manual, complete course, test papers, notes & pendulum   Accredited & Certified
An enlightened & fascinating modality of healing brought forward from Atlantean teachings, using kinesiology, colour therapy, Gem Essences, and circular polarisation of energy through crystals. Students will work with a client to locate and balance energy flow disturbances to the 14 major organs. Locate & balance the emotions creating the energy blockage. Have a working knowledge of Chinese 5 elements, Ch'i flow, colour associated with each organ and it's healing properties, 18 Gem Essences & how to perform accurate muscle tests. A tool for many Kinesiologists. You will be able to practice professionally by the end of this day if desired.

Educational, fun, informative, Develop a new skill or expand on those you already have in health, healing and esoteric studies with the Crystal Light Balancing Course. Study in your own time, Set your own pace, Expand on skills for your own health, wellbeing and personal development as well as assisting those around you

Learn: how to utilise, practice & understand Basic Kinesiology (Muscle Testing), Learn: how to tap into your subconscious with the use of a Crystal Pendulum, Perform a Complete Chromotherapy Balance, Discover the Chinese theory of the 5 elements & how they can influence us in our day to day life, Understand some basic Crystallography, Delve into the subconscious emotional states that may be causing energy blockages & release these emotions, Learn about the Healing properties of Gem Essences & how to utilise them to add strength to your balance, Putting it all into a practical working order - Chromotherapy, Kinesiology, Pendulums, Emotional States, Gem Essences, Chakras, Meridian, Acupressure / Acupuncture Points & energy centres in the body.

Renascent Crystal Light Balancing
Color Therapy – Chromotherapy – Color Puncture

A perfect tool for Kinesiologists and natural therapists to use in their clinics and healing practices. Or for those interested in health maintenance of themselves and their family.

Crystal Light Balancing Advanced Color Healing

<u>HOW TO USE THE TORCH</u> By placing the appropriate color disc in the torch and either running this color along the appropriate meridian or holding it over the appropriate Acupressure Holding Points or Chakra. Energy will be assisted to flow through these areas and balance will be achieved. For Kinesiologists you may muscle test as to which points are out of balance to determine where the torch is needed. There are also gem essences and negative & positive emotions associated with each meridian and by locating these you will add depth and strength to your balance. Please refer to the Crystal Light Balancing Workbook for further information.. This referral is also necessary for those who do not know where the meridians are located on the body as well as locating a wide range of emotional imbalances that could be creating deeper concerns for your patient. **To insert color discs into torch**, slide plastic tip off with thumb, don't pull on crystal or twist. Drop disc in, replace on torch.

<u>ABOUT THE TORCH</u> A stunning healing modality tool, these specially designed color torches are of the highest quality, specifically made with integrity for use by natural therapists. The crystal tip is made of <u>natural</u>, uncut and unpolished Australian Quartz crystal, <u>double terminated and hand collected crystal</u> whenever possible. Hand selected for their energies and ease of refraction. The globe is a specific type to produce <u>perfect white light</u> thus ensuring your colors are not distorted, giving clarity and purity.

Basic Color Discs in set: (Use torch without a disc to produce white light)
RED ORANGE YELLOW GREEN BLUE VIOLET INDIGO
Advanced Color Discs in set: (Use torch without a disc to produce white light) ORCHID OCEANIC MIDNIGHT CHARCOAL RUBY HOLOGRAPHIC

TROUBLE SHOOTING & SPARE PARTS

My torch won't work: Firstly check the batteries are facing the correct direction; if this still doesn't work try replacing the globe. Located in the end of your torch is a spare globe. Locate the spring & carefully remove, you will find the globe behind this. It is imperative that you DO NOT TOUCH it with your skin. Wear gloves or use tweezers to remove & replace it. The oil on your skin can cause it to blow immediately. If this doesn't work, return the torch to where you purchased it. Batteries & globe will need to be replaced occasionally. Spare globes are available from Mag lite (ensure they are halogen globes) or directly from Renascent

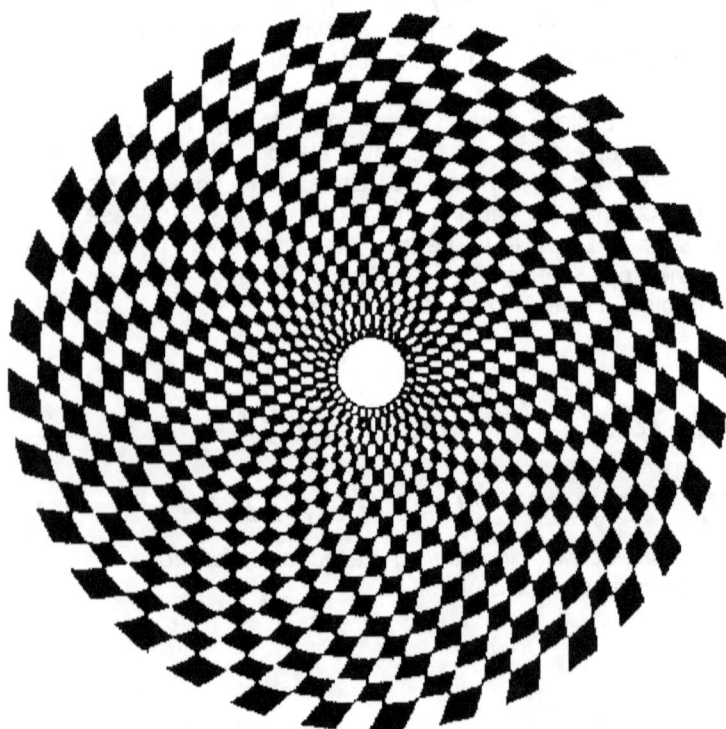

Auric Healing Color wheel

Hold this paper out in front of you around 30cm – 5 feet away & gaze into the center of the wheel.
Soon the pattern will begin to move and reflect with your auric colors

Your auric color(s) may change due to many effects including healing, negative situations, emotional states & as we progress on our life path, we may progress through events & develop a new state of being
It is excellent to have your patients stare at this wheel & explain the colors to you before and after a healing – they will generally notice some differences which you may explain to them as the energies becoming more harmonious.

Healing energies of the Crystal Light Balancing Advanced Color Healing Discs

Orchid – A wonderfully ethereal healing. The Orchid disc assists the patient to open their mind and uplift themselves to a higher level, especially beneficial to be utilised around the third eye to open to the angelic realms.

Orchid assists to release past hurts and allow the patient to realise their own beautiful nature. It assist you to feel comfortable with yourself and develop a strong sense of self love. Perfect for those who always place others needs before their own. By allowing the patient to realise their own beauty it also assists to realise their own importance in the world and their deep connection to spirit. Excellent for those who feel they have lost their way and need heavenly reconnection.

Oceanic – A beautifully serene form of color healing, Oceanic awakens energies of the ocean, including dolphin healing & allows the mind to stretch to new possibilities. Perfect when beginning new business opportunities & endeavours to allow the patient to see a wider picture and many ideas may now begin to be formulated that were previously overlooked. The ocean is ever-changing & from a distance appears to be stable. Yet on closer inspection we discover unpredictability, sensitivity, and power. This is similar to the human psyche & if we utilise the Oceanic disc it can represent our inner landscapes. When utilising the Oceanic healing, it may be beneficial to request your patient mentally bring this deep ocean imagery into their mind to assist in bringing deeper issues & emotions to the surface to heal during the balance. Once they have achieved this imagery, continue on with the balancing procedure passing the Oceanic color waves over the entire body, ask the patient to think of the sun, the sand, deep azure seas and any other elements that offer you guidance. In awakening these energies during the balance you will be assisting them to remove any negativity and reestablish emotional equilibrium.

Similar to the ocean's tides washing over the shores, removing debris & restoring balance, so can your Oceanic healing cleanse the soul of that which no longer serves us. As our daily life generally impacts upon us and brings negativity on a daily basic it is excellent to receive this Oceanic balance at least once a month.

Midnight – Assists to release & uplift negativity, fear, anxiety, hatred, resentment, guilt, & depression. It is excellent for grounding energies & allowing the patient to see their reason to live.

Providing a healing utilising the midnight disc gives the patient spiritual protection (especially beneficial if they are under psychic attack or entity attachment) whilst allowing them to feel independent, secure & safe. The midnight disc deepens our connection to all things physical, (the natural being). Whilst removing fears, especially those associated with our physical existence here on earth.

Midnight healing acts as a shield to protect and deflect negative energies that may come to you. At the same time it is beneficial for patients who do not like the way they look to bring a sense of self-acceptance.

The midnight discs brings a sense of being assertive, daring, intriguing, mysterious and independent... It allows the patient to feel grounded, confident, and fearless. Try it!

If your patient has been suffering from a depletion of energies (even after a holographic healing), utilise midnight to banish these negative energies.

(*As midnight & charcoal are similar in appearance, we have added a small circle to the midnight disc to distinguish them. As this is on the outside of the disc it will not affect your healings in any way)

Charcoal – Assists Spiritual healing. When the patient is suffering from a lack of commitment, or has depression of any form, utilise charcoal to uplift and remove these negative states of being. The Charcoal disc represents the energy of neutrality. It clears confusion and is of benefit when the patient feels that are out of balance or at a crossroads in life. When they are suffering from general depression or sadness, Charcoal will provide energy and guidance for problems/ situations that are arising.

Assists to heighten intuition and brings encouragement & support. Like midnight – it can be utilised to remove negativity and bring about hope, unconditional love, nurturing, grounding, a sense of appreciation of women and nature. It has been found to evoke mystic visions, spiritual and romantic love, tenderness, kindness, sensitivity and psychic abilities. Charcoal encourages stability; whilst assisting to develop psychic abilities with psychic protection.

To use: *you can pendulum, dowse or muscle test the most appropriate method of use for them. However I usually just apply the appropriate colour light into the forehead / third eye chakra and allow the energies to filter down throughout the body.*

Ruby – Assists to bring back a burning desire, a passion for life & the ability to regain drive, determination & creative energies. On a darker healing spectrum than the standard red disc, Ruby awakens deep desires and assists the patient to remember their life path & direction in life. Similar to red, Ruby heals unresolved emotions, particularly those in relation to a father figure, however with this healing comes an awakening of personal energies. Excellent for those who are feeling 'stuck in a rut', unable to complete projects or lost in their life direction. Excellent for any sluggish concerns within the body to move quickly through them and bring rapid healing. Often patients return home after a ruby healing and suddenly 'spring clean' & become involved in past projects that had been shelved (sometimes for years)

Holographic – Assists to heal damaged etheric energies. Hold over & move in a gentle circular motion over any area of the body that has been damaged to assist in 'knitting' the etheric back together. When the skin / organs are damaged often an energy breakage occurs allowing energy to leak out in a similar way to blood leaking out from a cut. Over time, left untreated this causes an energy depletion and renders the patient tired, lacking in energy / motivation, feeling lethargic, vague aches & pains and many other symptoms. By knitting the etheric back together with the holographic disc the energy breakage is healed and the patient is thus able to maintain their own energy levels. Often patients report an increase in energy, health & general well being simply by the use of this color therapy. As a complete balancing procedure, have you patient lay down and gently go over the entire body utilising the holographic disc. (If you think back over a lifetime of cuts, bruises & damage done to the body you will begin to realise how many of these energy breakages may be present). At the end of the session, your patient will be able to maintain energy throughout the entire body from this point on and should generally experience a better state of being almost immediately.

From this point onwards, the holographic disc can be utilised any time the body is damaged to maintain energetic health.

It is interesting to note that I have observed when viewed in standard light the light coming from the CLB tip (with the holographic disc inserted) seems to be just white light, yet if viewed in a darkened situation you are able to see the light refracting into several directions showing the varied energy axis & the 'meshing' of energies that takes place.

NATURAL THERAPIES COLLEGE – INC' CORRESPONDENCE COURSES

INTRODUCTORY EVENINGS & WORKSHOPS TO DIPLOMAS & MASTER CLASSES OR INSTRUCTOR TRAINING. IN PERSON & CORRESPONDENCE.

STUDY FOR FUN, PERSONAL DEVELOPMENT OR TO **WORK FOR YOURSELF IN A CAREER YOU LOVE:** All classes are accredited & most classes are professionally certified towards diplomas. In person or correspondence – you may begin your studies at any time.

THEY INCLUDE THESE MAIN STREAMS OF QUALIFICATIONS:

REIKI: A gentle, loving, non invasive form of healing. Perfect to utilise with massage or as a stand alone modality. From Western Usui system to the more traditional Japanese Reiki.

QI GONG: Gentle, yet powerful exercises to harmonise & enhance Ch'i which can be utilised for personal / spiritual development, healing abilities, martial arts & increased health

KINESIOLOGY: An important modality for anyone interested/working in any modality of natural health. As well as rebalancing & repatterning the body & mind, Kinesiology (muscle testing) will provide skills to verify the most appropriate oils/supplements/modality to use/etc. It will provide a physical change which you/your clients can experience for themselves. There will be dramatic differences in the body's relative strength before and after balancing & provides a more tangible modality to use with energy work. We recommend this course to all healers & health workers. a natural approach to restoring our natural energies, health using acupressure, ancient teachings, touch and massage.

NATURAL HEALTH SCIENCES: A rounded, well balanced choice of study offering many different topics. Perfect for those who wish to utilise a variety of healing modalities or as a 'taster' course to determine your best areas of interest. Inc: Crystal Light Balancing, Crystals, EMF's, Gem & Stellar Essences, Healing, Meditation, Tien Ti, Craft, Anatomy.

CRYSTALS: basic & some advanced principles of crystal healing - Chakra balancing, Auric Alignments, Choosing a crystal, Cleansing, Healing, Harmonising, Electromagnetic fields & their effects.

GEM ESSENCES: Manufacture of gem essences, Natural Healing, Practitioner advice, In depth healing, geological & mythological properties of over 40 gems and crystals, Usage of essences. + **TRAINING AS AN INSTRUCTOR**: To teach the gem essence certificate course,

CRYSTAL LIGHT BALANCING & Color Therapy: A powerful tool for natural therapists & body workers, utilising color, crystal healing, emotions, meridians and gem essences to heal and rebalance your physical body, thoughts and emotions - create health serenity and wellbeing.

FENG SHUI & GEOMANCY: Utilised by many health workers, architects, builders & interior designers. Discover how to work in harmony with the unseen energies in our homes, businesses & environments. Improve your home or train as a professional consultant. The Chinese art of placement. This ancient art not only makes your environment more pleasant and harmonious to be in, on a deeper level it contains all the secrets to everything that is going on around you. Could it be true that your house determines your destiny and vice versa?

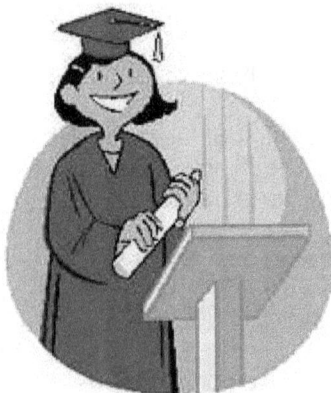

GEOMANCY: Hand in hand with Feng Shui, explore ancient divination methods. Ley Lines, psychic impressions, Omphalos points in the environment, discover how your house may boost or hinder your health.

PERSONAL DEVELOPMENT: Spiritual Development classes, Vegetarian Cooking, eBay - beginners to advanced business selling, Melt & Pour Soap Making to advanced soap art 'works of art' - through to fabulous journeys overseas. Fun, Hobbies, Personal Awakening & all great sharing!

All Seminars are taught by highly experienced facilitators, specialists in their chosen field(s).

RENASCENT NEW AGE PRODUCTS - RETAIL & WHOLESALE

Renascent stock a wonderful range of new age and alternative therapies products, Retail & Wholesale catalogues available

SOME OF THE PRODUCTS AVAILABLE INCLUDE:

GEM ESSENCES: One of the purest & most potentised gem essence ranges in the world with the most comprehensive training system available. Also Pure Aromatherapy Oils naturally diffused with Gem Essences.

BOOKS, FULL COLOR WALL CHARTS & POSTERS - On crystals, Gem Essences, Feng Shui, Aromatherapy, Herbalism, Manuals, Workbooks, Color Therapy, Crystal Moonlight Runes.

FENG SHUI PRODUCTS & SYMBOLS: to improve Ch'i flow

NATURAL CRYSTAL PENDULUMS, CHROMOTHERAPY TORCHES, BOOKS & ESSENCES: For Color Therapy

CH'I ENERGY PRODUCTS: Electromagnetic & psychic protection, Increase energy, motivation and personal unfoldment.

STELLAR ESSENCES: A new and powerful form of vibrational healing.

GEMS & CRYSTALS: A wide variety of common & unusual specimens.

YOU ARE SURE TO BE DELIGHTED AT THE HIGH INTEGRITY & SUPPORT OF OUR PRODUCTS. All Products are available for purchase by mail order

Renascent Crystal Light Balancing Course

An enlightened & fascinating modality of healing brought forward from Atlantean teachings, using kinesiology, colour therapy, Gem Essences, and circular polarisation of energy through crystals. Students will work with a client to locate and balance energy flow disturbances to the 14 major organs. Locate & balance the emotions creating the energy blockage. Have a working knowledge of Chinese 5 elements, Ch'i flow, colour associated with each organ and it's healing properties, 18 Gem Essences & how to perform accurate muscle tests. One of the common tools of many Kinesiologists.You will be able to practice professionally by the end of this course.

Color therapy, Kinesiology, Pendulums, Chinese 5 elements, deep emotional balancing.
An exciting powerful & deeply aligning natural therapy correction. For beginners & practitioners alike

Renascent Crystal Light Balancing Gem Essences

The gem essence kit is designed to work with the Crystal Light Balancing manual (Book) & seminar, however it may be used alone. The kit contains 20 pure stock strength (not dilutions) gem essences especially chosen to rebalance emotions that cause meridian imbalance. All essences and their appropriate use for each meridian are listed in the Renascent Crystal Light Balancing Workbook. A beautiful method of healing & bringing back clarity and a feeling of greater empowerment.

Renascent Crystal Light Balancing Torch

Complete in a sturdy carry case, with: Torch (batteries, clip & spare globe) Halogen globes, Quartz Crystal tip and 7 color discs. 4 for the Renascent Crystal Light Balancing & an extra 3 (no additional charge) for Chakric work. The color gels are a particular shade that produces balance in the energy systems.

ABOUT THE TORCH A stunning new healing modality tool, specially designed torches of the highest quality, specifically made with integrity for use by natural therapists. The crystal tip is made of natural, uncut and unpolished Australian Quartz crystal. Hand selected for their energies and ease of refraction. The globe is halogen to produce perfect white light thus ensuring your colors are not distorted for effective healing.

HOW TO USE THE TORCH By placing the appropriate color disc in the torch and either running this color along the appropriate meridian or holding it over the appropriate Acupressure Holding Points. Energy will be assisted to flow through these areas and balance will be achieved. Kinesiologists may muscle test which points are out of balance to determine where the torch is needed. By utilising CLB gem essences & negative & positive emotions associated with each meridian, add depth and strength to your balance.

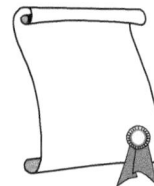

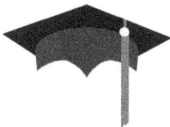

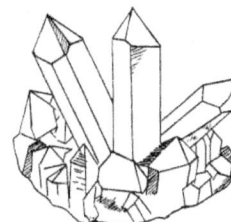

CRYSTAL LIGHT BALANCING &
CHROMOTHERAPY WORKBOOK

Published by - Renascent
First Published in 1994, revised & reprinted in 2004, 2009, 2016

AUSTRALIAN NATIONAL LIBRARY

Cataloguing-in-Publication-Entry
Mitchell (nee Antonoff) Lesley, Keele-
bedford Denise
Crystal Light Balancing & Chromotherapy
Workbook
I.S.B.N. 978-0-646-20830-5

Renascent
143 Research-Warrandyte Rd,
Warrandyte Nth 3113
Australia
Website: www.renascentcollege.com or www.RenascentbathBody.com.au

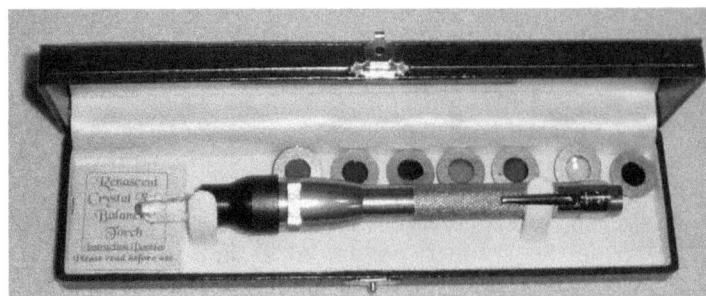

PERFECT FOR BEGINNERS AND ADVANCED NATURAL THERAPISTS ALIKE

Uncovering an exciting new healing modality
Explore Color Puncture (Chromotherapy)

Book Contents

* Circular Polarisation of light and energy to sweep heaviness from the mind, body and emotions
* Color Therapy and spiral energy flows
* Ancient healing techniques dating back to Tibetan monks
* Meridians and Acupressure Holding Points
* Crystal Pendulums - Can you use this ancient divining tool ?
* Qi or Chi flow within the body - would you like greater vitality, More energy, better health and an increased zest for life
* Gem Essences - to harmonise, balance and create serenity and inner peace - understand basic crystallography
* Emotional states that can lead to imbalances in the body and how to improve and correct the energy flow to them
* Kinesiology (Muscle Testing) correction pages
* Step by step instructions to inform, entice and assist you
* Treat yourself, friends and family to health through increased energy flow and harmonised emotions
* Discover the Chinese theory of the 5 elements & how they can influence us in our day to day life
* Perform a Complete Chromotherapy Balance
* Delve into the subconscious emotional states that may be causing energy blockages & release these emotions
* Learn about the Healing properties of Gem Essences & how to utilise them to add strength to your balance
* Putting it all into a practical working order - Chromotherapy, Kinesiology, Pendulums, Emotional States, Gem Essences
* Chakras, Meridian, Acupressure / Acupuncture Points & energy Centres in the body

Learned so much - taught with love and care

Comments from Renascent students

One of the simplest yet most powerful forms of natural therapy I have discovered

Course hours are accredited towards the Diploma of Natural Health Sciences. & the Certificate of Professional Kinesiology Consultant with Renascent & The International College of Intuitive Sciences

Very illuminating - learnt lots

A simple modality of healing able to be learnt by anyone and those around them with a desire to help themselves

A wonderful new form of therapy embodying centuries old techniques

Wonderful, worthwhile, tremendous eye opener

Lesley Mitchell is the author of 9 books, an international lecturer, natural therapist, Kinesiology, Gem Essence & Crystal Workshop Instructor. Lesley holds diplomas in Metaphysics, Spiritualism, Kinesiology, Feng Shui, Geomancy and Gemmology and has been teaching natural energy techniques & gemmology since 1988. Lesley is the founder of Renascent & co director of The International College of Intuitive Sciences.
Www.renascentcollege.com